Y0-AWH-783

BIRTH OF A FAMILY

BIRTH
OF A FAMILY

A Preparation for Parenthood

DR. CLAIR ISBISTER

HAWTHORN BOOKS, INC.
Publishers/NEW YORK
A Howard & Wyndham Company

BIRTH OF A FAMILY

Copyright © 1978, 1976 by Clair Isbister. Copyright under International and Pan-American Copyright Conventions. All rights reserved, including the right to reproduce this book or portions thereof in any form, except for the inclusion of brief quotations in a review. All inquiries should be addressed to Hawthorn Books, Inc., 260 Madison Avenue, New York, New York 10016. This book was manufactured in the United States of America.

This book was first published in Australia by Thomas Nelson and Sons Ltd.

Library of Congress Catalog Card Number: 78-52878

ISBN: 0-8015-0653-0

2 3 4 5 6 7 8 9 10

To my husband, James,
whose love, tolerance, strength, and personal
integrity have made my work possible and set
standards that I have tried to reach.

Contents

Acknowledgments

Apart from the acknowledgments made to the literature in the bibliography, I should like to say how grateful I am to a number of people who have greatly influenced me, some met only occasionally, since they are spread over the world: Dr. Mavis Gunther, Professor Niles Newton, Dr. W. G. Whittlestone, Dr. Ronald Mackeith, Professor W. Barclay—all of whose writings have been an inspiration, all of whom accept nothing without exposing it to the hard, bright light of scientific truth, all of whom love their fellow man and care where he is going. I also want to thank Dr. Grace Browne and the late Professor F. J. Browne, who gave constant encouragement, and Dr. Elaine McKinnon, Dr. Joan Thomas, and Dr. Jean Benjamin, with whom I have thrashed out many doubts and discussed the needs of mothers.

My thanks also go to Alison Quinn, my niece, for help with diagrams, and to my secretary, Beverley Pye, for endless typing and retyping.

I am grateful to Ross Laboratories (Columbus, Ohio) for allowing me to reproduce several pictures from their booklets on child care.

C.I.

BIRTH OF A FAMILY

Introduction

The Changing Scene

It is ten years since my book *Preparing for Motherhood* first appeared, and though there have been minor revisions and reprints, so much has happened in those ten years that I now need to write a new book to say what I want to say. The changes are not so much medical as social, though there have been considerable changes in the management of childbirth that husbands and wives will want to understand. In *Preparing for Motherhood* I dived straight into the signs of pregnancy in the second paragraph and cheerfully advanced through pregnancy and labor; I saved some philosophizing for the end and rather apologetically suggested that a little more thought given to the meaning of marriage might make everyone happier. But times have changed. A greater number of girls become pregnant before marriage; some 70 percent of the girls under twenty having their first baby conceive it out of wedlock; about half of these do get married, but many, of this group particularly, decide within two years that they have made a mistake and get divorced.

The divorce rate has risen to one in two in California and one in four in parts of Australia. Abortions have become easier to get as a result of alterations in the interpretation of the law and changes in the laws throughout the world, such as the British Abortion Act and the pronouncement of the United States Supreme Court. In Australia medical abortionists have appeared on TV advertising their clinics and have circularized the medical profession. Some active members of Family Planning Associations, which receive government support to the tune of hundreds of thousands of dollars annually, have supported abortion clinics to meet the world problem of overpopulation. The International Planned Parenthood Federation now holds international conferences of a very high standard. The Roman Catholic church has a large section rebelling against papal condemnation of the pill, and some very efficient scientific work is being done on ovulation control and ovulation awareness for those who prefer natural if less reliable methods of population control. So I must now include a chapter on contraception, family planning, and abortion. Zero Population Growth and Erlich have toured the world!

Women's liberation, with Greer, Millett, and Friedan demanding women's rights but often denying their womanhood, has thoroughly confused some women about their role. Women have returned to paid employment in ever-increasing numbers. Gay liberation has emerged to claim as normal some expressions of human sexuality that are, to say the least, sterile. Sex education in schools has become a big issue the world over; and in some countries, America and Scandinavia for instance, the teaching of physical facts without moral and ethical guidance seems to have had the same effect as the campaign against fires: It made so many people think about fires that more got lit. The increase in sexual activity among teen-agers may also be associated with the wide use of sexually seductive themes in advertising and of explicit and deviant material in the theater, in films, and on TV, so that the adolescents are finding it difficult to know what is normal and to distinguish between biological sexual attraction and the meaningful relationship with total personality involvement needed to make a success of marriage with its long-term commitment to partner and children. In fact, we have almost seen a reversal of norms, with marriage regarded by some of the young and the disillusioned as an outdated institution.

Individual freedom to "do one's own thing" is the catchcry of the times, and we must all welcome the widespread acceptance of the importance of the individual; but freedom carries responsibilities, and in the midst of all this "liberty" in a rapidly changing world, millions of children are growing up trying to establish for themselves standards by which to run their lives, trying to find out what they want from life without understanding what they will need to put into it. Only too often doing one's own thing is doing what the peer group is doing, not developing one's own individuality. Dr. Stanley Gold, addressing an international conference of psychiatrists, said, "The new freedoms seem to lead not to maturity, peace and love but to an increasing lack of concern for individuals . . . toward an unfeeling corporate structure." The poet Phyllis McGinley, while recognizing woman's right to fight for recognition as a person, said of the radical women's libber,

> *Snugly upon the equal heights*
> *Enthroned at last where she belongs,*
> *She takes no pleasure in her Rights*
> *Who so enjoyed her Wrongs.*

It may take strong action to obtain the rights that all women should have, but clearing the way to equal pay and equal opportunity in the work force does not necessarily enable a woman to lead a more satisfying life. True liberation is more than opening gates; it involves learning how to use one's liberty, removing fear, knowing oneself and one's potential and how to develop it, learning how to live with others and respect their liberty and rights.

In a society such as ours that has a morbid fear of death and illness, that consumes incredible amounts of pills and proprietary medicine, and is turning to the occult and Eastern mystics in search of truth, there are many people trying to escape from reality, filling their lives with trivialities, and indulging in the gratification of primal urges that brings little joy as they exploit others. But I have great confidence in the basic good sense of people and their desire to do what is good. I was struck by another statement of Dr. Gold's: "To mistake good for bad may lead to neurosis, to mistake bad for good is to become confused, perverted and mad." My many years of talking with parents and young people have confirmed me in my belief that they seek to know what is good for them and their families: They look for information that will enable them to understand what is happening to them and their community, and they will adapt that knowledge to their lives.

Most young couples still choose to marry and 80 percent choose to be married with a religious ceremony, taking what they mean to be a lifelong pledge; and even most of those having registry office weddings accept the family way of life as their aim. As I listen day by day in my consulting room to stories of emotional and physical illness in children, aggravated and even caused by unhappy and broken families, I have come to realize more and more how important the family is. But the family does need emancipating from the stereotyped sex roles that have dominated it in the past. It now has to meet the needs of all its members; no member must be sacrificed to it anymore. It delights me to find that whereas years ago mothers brought their children to me themselves or with grandmother, now father accompanies mother as often as not. Father has really entered into the everyday living of the family that functions well, but he needs a lot more knowledge of his new role and he deserves a lot more attention to his needs.

The increasing number of children in one-parent families, or in families in which only one parent is their own, fills me with deep sorrow when I think of what my parents meant to me and how devastating it would have been for me and my children had I had to rear them without their father.

As I write this book my great desire has been to communicate some of the knowledge gained from research and to indicate some of the ways of finding joy and fulfillment in the intimate relationships the family can provide and some of the ways in which the hazards and tragedies can be avoided or mastered. In communities that can read and write, or even just see and hear with TV, radio, and tape recorders, it should be possible to give men and women some of the knowledge that can help to a more satisfying life. Communication is full of problems, and here I am trying honestly to use words to communicate accurate scientific knowledge, actual experiences and feelings. Some will have trouble with the words. If you favor the Anglo-Saxon terms (euphemistically known as four-letter words) used by some primary school children, uneducated adults, and mixed-up academics, you won't find them here, because I do not believe in debasing the written language. Some will think I push a point, but I am only pushing to keep the family and the standards of human behavior on the right road.

Let's not just think about pregnancy and childbirth and physical facts. Let's think about the family as the fundamental unit of society: man, woman, and child as a flexible, functioning unit. The best way to bring up children is in the family group, and I hope this book, as well as being a guide in preparing for motherhood, may help to stimulate the cooperation between man and woman that is so necessary from the beginning.

1

The Nuclear Family

The family is coming in for a lot of criticism these days. Within a few weeks I have heard a cleric speaking in a court of the Presbyterian church say that the family is out of date, a young communist declaring that communes where the children are pooled and the sex partners shared is the ideal, and a pair of ornately garbed hippies with their child shout "Down with the nuclear family!" at a public meeting. In my medical practice I meet women rearing children without fathers; I meet others in *de facto* relationships that they say are easier to get out of than a marriage if the relationship does not work; I meet young couples living on the salary of one, determined that their child shall not be deprived of its mother for a moment, even though the father has to work overtime to keep her at home; I meet mothers who leave their young babies with baby-sitters all day and are determined that nothing will interfere with their careers; and now and again I meet a man who stays at home and cares for the child while the mother works. There is no doubt that a great deal of thinking and talking is going on about the family; and the *nuclear family* is a term used scornfully by many young moderns who say we must do away with it. I want to preserve and strengthen it.

What Is the Nuclear Family?

The nuclear family is father, mother, and their offspring—the two-generation unit that is the basic unit of our society, described in the Universal Declaration of Human Rights of the United Nations as the "natural and fundamental group unit of society and entitled to protection by society and the state." A little wider and more a legal definition is that used in *Beyond the Best Interests of the Child* (Joseph Goldstein, Anna Freud, and Albert Solnit): "The intimate group of adults and their children constitute the central core of a family. Responsibility for the child, for his survival, for his physical and mental adaptation to community standards, becomes that of designated adults in a family to whom the child in his turn is responsive and accountable"—usually parents, whether biological or adoptive.

I have heard the poor New York family defined as "a man, a woman purporting to be his wife, 1.27 children, and 2 social workers"; no doubt the decimal fraction decreased with the abortion rate! The nuclear family sadly familiar to so many is more aptly described as I heard a young man from a broken family put it recently: "one battle after another, finally ending in an almighty explosion with everyone hurt in the fallout." So devastating has been the explosion for many that it is small wonder they cannot believe that good families exist, and therefore want to try another pattern and experiment with dangerous alternatives.

Our affluent society seems to have so much to offer a child—health, education, material comforts, a wide choice of careers, mobility to explore the world, leisure, and a degree of social security unknown to our forebears. Why is it becoming increasingly difficult to give a child what all the experts in child welfare, both educators and psychologists, say matters most all through life—a stable family, parents who care about him and give him love, guidance, and appropriate protection from the dangers that threaten as he grows up and is prepared for life's journey? Why is it difficult to get parents who will stay with him and accept commitment to the family? Why are an increasing number of children being reared in one-parent families? The emphasis these days is on the quality of life, yet "there can be conditions for children amounting to an emotional slum in situations of prestige and material plenty" (Parker). Michael Davie, writing in the *Sunday Observer* about life in affluent California, said, "I began to feel that I had seen the future and it did not work." Toffler in *Future Shock* has given a frightening picture of the mobile family with the father more mobile than the rest of the unit, even suggesting that as he moves around the country he needs alternative families to connect with in a wife-swapping arrangement to meet the sexual needs of both. Perhaps, as some say, it really is the effluent society! The nuclear family is certainly experiencing a high breakdown rate that is heart-breaking; but it is the children who suffer most, and we must consider what can be done, what alternatives there are.

Need for a Social Group

Every animal that shares this world with us has needed a social group for evolution and survival. In many animals the young have needed a constant adult for survival and succesful rearing; this has usually been the mother and in mammals lactation has firmly secured the mother-child bond. While the mother gives birth to her baby, nurtures it, and teaches it how to find its own food and protect itself, the group offers some protection; she is part of the herd. In animal families the father often takes an active part in protecting his own mate and baby and in bringing them food. There are many patterns of survival in the animal kingdom whereby the young are protected from predators; but man, the supreme predator, has wiped out many species. It is to be hoped that he does not wipe out his own, for man himself is no exception in needing the family system for survival.

Man has existed mainly in tribes that have protected the mother-child relationship. The father does not always take direct responsibility for his child; sometimes it is his brother, or the whole tribe, that accepts responsibility. This may well have been an important factor in survival and emotional stability in fighting tribes, where the man had a short life-span; a child gains security with several men and women, but the blood relationship is always regarded as important. No doubt ownership of land and the acquisition of possessions tightened the family and made smaller groups. The banding together of whole tribes to make a country, pooling their defenses, by agreement or by conquest, allowed individual families to be better protected and the system took care of the family, even though many lived in poverty and were made to serve a master. Even in the more primitive tribes males and females had definite roles and the children learned their role.

With urbanization and civilization the family became more compact, but it was a three-generation family. A child had parents, grandparents, cousins, aunts, and uncles, and he knew them all. But there have been great wars, and Australia, America, and Canada all have been largely populated by migrant people transplanted from their culture, able to bring only some of it with them and often having retained only their compact, overstressed two-generation family. Democratically elected governments in these countries protect the welfare of the people and provide, to a varying degree, education, health services, and social welfare, and in so doing impose a pattern that may be different from the parents' cultural pattern. Socialist countries have more standardized patterns, but all still recognize that the child's own parents have rights and that the child has a right to his own family. To quote Sir James Spence, writing thirty years ago: "Does not human welfare depend on a recognition that the unit of human existence is not the isolated individual but the family?"

The Family Unit

At its best what does a family unit provide?

It meets the physical needs of the parents and children for housing, food, hygiene, disposal of waste, and an environment that provides protection, rest, and the conveniences of everyday living.

It provides protection and care for the pregnant woman and the mother while she cares for little children.

It provides the environment in which the child learns the pattern of everyday living, eating,and sleeping habits, hygiene, speech (all mainly learned by copying his parents, but with guidance and reminding). Here the child learns to live with others;

by loving and being loved and by learning self-discipline he learns how to master the green-eyed monster of jealousy and to love the new baby; he learns how to control anger and how to avoid arousing anger in others.

The child has protection and encouragement during times of stress such as illness, starting school, going to a hospital, separation from parents for increasing periods of time. He learns about being male and female, sex identification, and understanding of gender; he learns how men and women behave as he sees his mother and father manage their lives—better still if he sees aunts and uncles and grandparents—and subconsciously he accepts the pattern of family life they have set for him. The well-functioning family unit meets the need of the parents for love, emotional support, companionship; it meets their sexual needs and their need for encouragement and protected retreat in times of stress. It takes time, determination, caring concern for each other, and a lot of adjustment to develop a good team. We all have our bad days, but a child can accept those as he sees the relationship develop and strengthen. The family has also been the medium for passing on religious and cultural attitudes from one generation to the next.

An exhaustive search of the literature at the time I wrote *Mother on the Watch* for the World Health Organization's twenty-fifth anniversary showed me that there is still no more satisfactory arrangement for rearing children than to have a father and mother committed to their long-term care and to each other, and that love, tenderness, unselfishness, loyalty, mutual trust, and concern for each other's well-being provide the best atmosphere in which to learn to live. Research confirms that the well-functioning family can sustain its members in spite of terrible disasters, but there are families with such internal stresses that they cannot cope with even minor strains. The children in such families are in great danger, whether the families break up or precariously hang together, particularly if there is no larger family of grandparents, aunts, and uncles to cushion the trauma. Blood is still thicker than water, as even the sex-partner–swapping communes have found. No social services, cash handouts, or legally decreed child maintenance can ever repair the damage of a failed family. "If the family fails the other institutions which deal with the child face a tremendous, usually impossible, handicap" (Havighurst and Taba).

Three Types of Family

There are three main types of family in our Western society.

The best functioning is the one that permits individuality and recognizes each person's right to develop his own talents and be an individual while accepting his responsibility in the group; it meets the needs of the whole family and it also keeps contact with and to some extent takes responsibility for its "old folks." This type of family is a three-generation family; it faces reality well and can accept old age and death and the vicissitudes of life with reasonable equanimity; it has its ups and downs and at times life in it can be a stormy affair, but it maintains a stability and it cares about all its members.

The two-generation family is very vulnerable to stress and is often isolated. It may recognize the individuality of its members and their needs, but because of limited security and lack of the cultural background grandparents can give it makes very heavy demands on its members and lacks the safety valve of other blood relations.

The third type of family may be of two or three generations. It does not recognize the individual needs of its members; father and mother tend to follow fixed roles according to the code of behavior of their parents. "The children are your responsibility, dear. I bring home the money!" You know the setup. Members of such a family may follow the rules even of a religious code without adequately relating them to the reality of their everyday lives. This type of family has been held together by social pressure to preserve marriage in the past; it is breaking up now, and it sets unsatisfactory patterns for children whether it breaks up or not. To survive, a family must be able to adapt to change and appreciate the fundamental needs of its individual members.

Influences on the Family

The influences operating on the family from outside are now very strong and often uncontrolled. Past generations accepted that children needed special care, guidance, and protection from moral and physical harm, that men and women had complementary roles in marriage and society, that a child needed a male and female parent. It was accepted that prostitution, temporary or casual sexual relationships outside marriage, premarital sexual relationships in adolescence (at least for women), early sexual stimulation of children, and homosexual relationships all operated against the ability of a man and woman to establish the type of lasting relationship they need for the conditions in which to rear children. But attitudes to these forms of behavior are now in the melting pot, and TV programs coming into our homes present such situations as being normal. Parents are finding it very difficult to establish a family pattern for their children to follow or even to keep to one themselves. A few generations ago they had their children at home for six or seven years, but now the children are into the peer group by three and a half at kindergarten, and some even go into it at the day-nursery stage and grow up in it. A child's ability to cope with stress and his environment still depends basically on the parents' ability to adjust the environment in the early years and set him a pattern for living; but now the parents, too, have been buffeted by change. Consider how you are affected by the employment situation, your health,

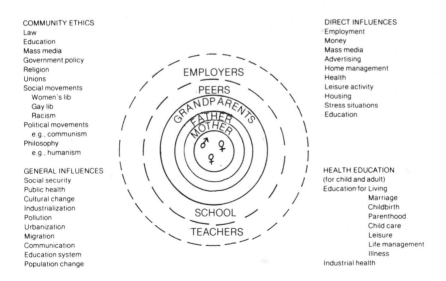

COMMUNITY ETHICS
Law
Education
Mass media
Government policy
Religion
Unions
Social movements
  Women's lib
  Gay lib
  Racism
Political movements
  e.g., communism
Philosophy
  e.g., humanism

GENERAL INFLUENCES
Social security
Public health
Cultural change
Industrialization
Pollution
Urbanization
Migration
Communication
Education system
Population change

DIRECT INFLUENCES
Employment
Money
Mass media
Advertising
Home management
Health
Leisure activity
Housing
Stress situations
Education

HEALTH EDUCATION
(for child and adult)
Education for Living
  Marriage
  Childbirth
  Parenthood
  Child care
  Leisure
  Life management
  Illness
Industrial health

Influences on the nuclear family

your housing, your recreational pleasures, and the unrelenting mass media telling you what the world is doing and trying to persuade you to buy! buy! buy! The peer group has in many cases become a stronger influence than the family, and its constant exposure to mass media is molding moral and social attitudes. This is particularly so if the central family group breaks and the child has to seek emotional support elsewhere.

The peer-group culture is not an ideal one. Even the kibbutz that has been acclaimed as the best family substitute is now being examined by psychiatrists as the children, grown to adults, start their own families. Bettelheim observed less psychiatric disturbance, less neglect, better education, but more conformity, less individuality, less adventurous thinking, less creativity, and a loss of ability to form close relationships; the kibbutz was not ideal, but it was certainly better than a bad family environment. Many are arguing that this is what we need in the new world, people who do not get involved, people who are satisfied with casual relationships, but these are usually people who find they have no aim. In Russia, China, and Israel we have seen a people working for a cause, and this cannot be compared with what we see in our culture, where immediate self-gratification now seems to be the primary aim.

We recognize that most of the social problems in our society are associated with family instability. We have even seen a breakdown to a family that is just mother and child; here the involvement is too intense and the possibility of neglect or failure to meet the child's needs too great. Even in the nuclear family, when father is still there, he may be away so much that mother and child are together too much. Dr. John Bowlby says that "it is a monstrous insult to expect a woman with young children to go to work"; but he also says it is "very unnatural for a woman to be cooped up with a baby for twelve hours a day."

Psychology and psychiatry have much to answer for with their emphasis on the individual and sex. Sex and violence have taken over the film and TV screens. They have changed the social norms as they enter every household. Computers are gobbling up statistics and spitting out correlations for research workers; but while many films display the joys of physical sex as early as possible, it is very difficult to get publicity for a study showing that successful marriage correlates best with premarital chastity, and that of those college girls seeing psychiatrists 70 percent had had premarital sexual experience as against 22 percent in the total female college population.

Women searching for individuality, whether they go to work or stay at home, are confused and anxious. The role of wife and mother is not prestigious or economically profitable and its main attackers are now those extremists in the women's liberation movement who launch their main offensive against traditional sexual morality and in so doing are further breaking up the family. It is all very well to demand equal opportunity and rewards and to attack the double sexual standards of behavior, but we do not raise women's prestige by trying to tear down the achievements of men or improve relationships by taking over their role. Some of the aggressive, violent women among the liberationists are not suited to caring for children. Others, hurt by divorce or let down by men who promised so much, are defiantly proving that they can go it alone; but they and their children suffer.

Male and Female Qualities

In the new family pattern father and mother are both very involved in family care but still have their male and female role to play. I once heard a little girl call the preparation for parenthood classes "classes for turning husbands and wives into daddies and mommies." How do you feel about becoming mommy and daddy? With the Greers and Milletts saying that maleness and femaleness are all conditioned anyway, and the women's lib writers of children's books sending Snow White down the mine with the dwarfs to reverse the awful process, you need to do some hard thinking. If prospective daddy always gets the newspaper and sits down in front of TV after dinner, leaving expectant mother with the dishes, then his conditioning is out of date; but if she makes a habit of spending the afternoon at the hairdresser or a show and buys him a pizza on the way home, then hers may not be too good either.

Failure to appreciate the fundamental differences between male and female attitudes to life is the cause of a great deal of misunderstanding in marriage, and you will find that many dissatisfied women and playboy men are either divorced or trying out temporary relationships that eventually break up. Men and women did not become conditioned to their roles accidentally. Nature's primary concern is continuation of the race and the care of the next generation so that it will survive to rear future generations: So woman has a womb where she cares for and protects and nurtures the baby until it is ready to breathe and survive outside the womb; and some experts in child care refer to the next nine months of close mother-child contact as the external womb. Nature provided the woman with breasts to make the ideal food, and hormones to go with them to make her accept her task with both joy and apprehension. Social change has increased the fear and reduced the joy because now she may not have the security of having learned the art and science of child care from her mother. She lacks confidence in her ability to care for a child. The contrast between her efficiency in the job she was trained for and her first efforts at baby care can be very demoralizing. Her education and experience have shown her that she can do almost any job a man can do and often do it better; she tends to reject man's protectiveness and even to regard it as patronizing superiority. Instead of accepting that male and female roles are different in parenthood, just as in procreation, and that protection of her is part of his role, she rejects his help. I have heard women say that they don't need one man, that they are not going to be tied, that they can give their child everything a man can—and they deprive the child of a parent.

Admittedly man and woman are basically different by only one chromosome in forty-six: She has XX and he has XY. The Y chromosome is just a little one and if there is anything wrong with the genes in it, or if his single X carries an abnormal gene (as for hemophilia or color blindness), we get a male sex-linked abnormality. The XX combination is likely to get these problems. Somehow the XY is associated with a greater predisposition to many illnesses and goes with a shorter life-span. Even as a baby a male is less likely to survive. Woman needs protection during her pregnancy and as she cares for young children, but she is the stronger at other times and her man needs her care.

The difference between the male hormone testosterone and the female estradiol is only four atoms of hydrogen and one of carbon, but just as every cell in the body is different with the chromosomes XX and XY, so the hormones affect the whole body too. The girl grows faster, speaks and gets teeth earlier, and is fully mature by twenty-one, whereas the boy will not be fully grown till twenty-four years. She ends up smaller than her comparable male relatives, her shape different with her wide pelvis for a baby to pass through and her breasts to feed him; even her hands and feet and arms and hips are different, and these physical differences put her at a disadvantage in running and throwing and she is not as strong as the comparably trained man. A woman's heart beats faster, she breathes faster, her body temperature is higher, but she can cool herself faster. In general, women have more acute senses of hearing, seeing, and feeling, and tolerate pain better (all scientifically proven). No doubt nature has equipped her better to detect danger when she cares for the young and to tolerate the discomfort of childbirth. The writer Randolph Stow in one of his novels describes a mother as "knowing an infinite number of ways of dying." We women all have good imaginations when it comes to danger threatening our children. When your husband retires to bed and appears to be at death's door and expects to be waited on hand and foot, then he really does feel bad, and you think he is worse! It's just good old Nature making sure you look after him, so don't resist her.

What if the hormones are out of balance? The castrated cat is not a very brave fellow; the castrated drake even loses the color in his feathers; the human who has both testicles or both ovaries removed before puberty does not grow normally, and the genitalia do not grow. It is only in the very early period while developing in the uterus—at about eight weeks—that the male and female look the same, and they look female; then, under the influence of the hypothalamus and male hormone, the male develops. The male is in general more aggressive; in the sad, terrible days when women with cancer of the breast were given male hormone injections in an effort to slow the cancer, I saw some of these women become aggressive viragoes, ruining their family's memories of them. Nature meant man to use his aggression to protect the woman and her child, to get food and keep away the enemy from his domain; but aggression is not all hormonal.

A psychologist-sociologist recently put forward the theory that now that man works away from home all day—in fact for weeks if he is a member of an air crew or a seaman or a salesman—then his place of work becomes his domain and he may transfer his sexual prowess to the office secretary or the air hostess; and his wife, left at home with the small children, has to adopt the protective role and mark out her area, so that she becomes more aggressive and militant. Watch some women in the supermarket or at a sale or even in the park and you will see how the modern world has changed them and why the traditional roles cannot be transferred into modern marriage. And what if mother is away at work too: Who protects the domain then?

The environment and the ways of living have certainly changed; but men and women were always different, and their hormones are different. Admittedly, some women have changed the balance of their hormones by using the contraceptive pills and having artificial menstrual periods and no ovulation. Scientists are watching this very carefully and most say that no harm results and that the situation is reversible; but others have observed subtle personality changes, often only really noticed by the husbands and often masked by the relief at avoiding pregnancy. Some women have already been subjected to such drastic cultural change in their upbringing that they do not know what the traditional family is or what family love and loyalty mean, and they find themselves in conflict with their hormones.

As one reads Germaine Greer's *The Female Eunuch* with its extraordinary, mixed-up psychology and elementary knowledge of physiology, endocrinology, and neurology, one realizes indeed that "a little learning is a dangerous thing" in the hands of one who can express herself so fluently and that such pseudoscience should be submitted to the brilliant light of truth, fact, and scientific criticism.

If theories are supposed to be based on science, then the science produced in their support must be accurate. Germaine Greer picks and chooses her science. I long ago learned to accept all research work with reservations until I knew something of the person doing it; it is incredibly easy to manipulate figures, and scientific research demands a standard of honesty that is not common. The dishonesty is not always conscious, and money, ambition, and sex are powerful influences.

We all have prejudices, firm beliefs, convictions—whatever we like to call them—that are deep-founded in our childhood and that subconsciously influence our actions. Love could not have figured much in Greer's childhood. I can sympathize with her great resentment of male domination and the exploitation of women. I can respect her mind and her mastery of English. But when she writes about babies and mother-child relationships and husband-wife relationships it seems to me that, through ignorance, she gravely distorts the picture. She plucks from odd bits of research what suits her argument; she quotes Freud to support her, then discards him when she disagrees with him. She sees the baby clutched in imprisoning hands as it emerges from the vagina; she sees its reflexes suppressed by swaddling clothes; she talks of the "intense absorption of the baby in one human being," the mother, as a relationship that increases in intensity until it becomes morbid and abnormal, instead of decreasing gradually to a relationship of equality and friendship. One wonders whether she has ever seen a baby born and put into the hands of its delighted mother, whether she has ever read Ribble or Middlemore or even the story of Harlow's monkey experiments. She seems to have no awareness of the need for emotional, social, and physical development to proceed together. She sees great virtue in babies being able to climb at eight months when experts are concerned about their being pushed to miss a stage like crawling, which now appears to be somehow concerned with speech.

Women have been listening to Germaine Greer and even believing her. But why accept the opinions on child-rearing and marriage of a woman who is prepared to kill her unborn child and abandon marriage in a few short weeks? What can she know of how to make a success of these most difficult and satisfying of women's roles? She has been given publicity and even encouraged to escape responsibility by the mass media, the sensation-seeking mass media that find news rather in what goes wrong than in what goes right.

In this confused age of unisex and superficial sex and homosex it becomes very necessary for scientifically trained people to try to counteract, then combat the insidious propaganda that threatens to destroy woman, the mother, and man, the father. It is not easy to gain an audience for sane views in a world that does not wish to hear them, and without the flamboyant use of four-letter words. *The Female Eunuch* has been a best seller while a book like *Childbearing—Its Social and Psychogenic Aspects* sits quietly on library shelves. Yet this book, originating from the Perinatal Research Committee of the United States, can demolish most of Greer's reference to the young and her theories on conditioning. Some women seem to want to ignore the emotional effects of hormones and deny the existence of the double XX, to abandon children and behave like a praying mantis devouring the male (Greer has even wrongly stated the number of chromosomes). Let us look at what that XX does: It produces woman, real woman, the lover emotionally as well as physically, bearing children, feeding them at her breast, being still the main guardian of their health, reveling in her femaleness, yet still woman the person.

Woman the person has rights and these too the world must recognize, the right to develop her talents, the right to identity and financial independence, the right to use and sell her talents in the community as a member of the work force, the right to be accepted as playing as important a part in the world as her male colleague, and the right to accept equal responsibility. The mistake of the liberationist is to regard herself as the center of the universe and put her interests before those of her child and her husband.

Margaret Mead has said that "where men have to want to be fathers, girls are committed by every cell in their bodies to be mothers." For normal women the creative urge is strong and insistent and difficult to deny. It is still the responsibility of the woman to give her child a father who wants to be a father and stay with them both and to keep him there. Men are more easily sexually aroused and more easily sexually satisfied than women. David Mace with his great experience in marriage counseling says that a man has more difficulty in expressing affection than a woman, but he wants her to understand and love him, not just be a sexual object; it is part of his masculinity to be able to satisfy a woman and be wanted by her. An American authority on marriage says that a man has arrived as a husband when he can say "I love you" in daylight and kiss his wife when it isn't necessary. Neither men nor women are finding full satisfaction in temporary relationships; women particularly find it very difficult to achieve in them the complete self-giving that makes full satisfaction possible. A woman feels secure only if the relationship is a committed one, or while she thinks it is, and one disillusionment may make the next relationship less satisfactory. A woman who has had a secure, happy family life with a good father-daughter relationship is most likely to have confidence in men. Sex in marriage is a progressively developing exclusive relationship if it is to be fully satisfying and endure; it is far more than physical pleasure, enjoyable though that can be.

Male and female are complementary roles, not equal or the same, but equally important. We need to appreciate each other's needs and differences, and to understand our dependence on each other. Usually it is men who fail in this, and many women in their frustration are demanding that the roles be similar and equal roles, and ruining the lives of their children.

I see more and more young men and women who do see their roles in the family as equally important. It is refreshing to meet so many fathers in the doctor's office these days, wanting to know what they must do for their wives and children. I have great hope for the family of the future, having the committed, exclusive, thoroughly satisfying relationships that are essential to the well-being of the race, having its ups and downs, but fully recognizing the equal but differing rights of man, woman, and child.

Nothing is achieved without having to overcome difficulties, so there must be difficulties to overcome. A very important part of the parents' role is to show a child how to overcome obstacles and threats to his security and to regulate the amount of stress the particular obstacle imposes on him at any particular time. There is no one less able to cope with life than the pampered girl who has always had all she wanted and never learned to control her mind, her emotions, her body, or her money. Since we are bound to be faced with some very changeable and erratic situations in our lives (as when stop–go governments and international crises throw people in and out of work), home should not be a peaceful, well-regulated place all the time. Parents do need to have a basic consistency in their management of their lives and of their children's behavior, but perfect calm does not help a child to cope with life, and an occasional blowup by mom or dad does no harm and perhaps some good. Some of the strongest characters in history have come from the most damaging backgrounds, and it was hardship that developed their strength; but in most, too, it developed a bitterness and ruthlessness that most of us do not want to see in our children. Perhaps our aim should be to regulate hardship, to impose some challenges, while seeing that emotional, social, physical, and educational needs are met.

The Need for a Government Policy

Though I am hopeful, I still fear for the nuclear family, and I think it will take a definite government policy of family encouragement to save it from further trouble. Governments in countries like Denmark, Sweden, and now Australia, which give the unmarried mother keeping her child more help than the mother who has committed herself to marriage and its responsibilities, are on dangerous ground. The family is the basic unit of society, and in any stable community the families of parents rearing their own children must make up the majority—or the next generation will suffer.

Governments must be prepared to strengthen the family by giving family concessions and services to make up for women having to give up their full-time jobs; more part-time work must be made available for women with families, and more part-time child-care facilities. Employers must provide this part-time work, and the public service should be setting the example. Employers should also be made to realize that sending men all over the country away from their families leads to family breakdown; shift work must make allowances for family needs. There must be more education for living. The educational system prepares children for the work force, not for life, and no wonder they are dropping out. Educational systems that glorify academic achievement and regard a college education as superior to a technical training must inevitably rob many people of one of their basic needs, the need to feel worthwhile in a worthwhile job. The illusion that it is a finer thing to be a professor of philosophy than a good plumber creates serious achievement problems in society. Everyone has talents and can use them in the right occupation to win the satisfaction and self-respect that achievement brings. The arts and crafts of everyday living should be subjects taught to all.

It is the duty of governments to strengthen and encourage the family pattern that is the basis of our society rather than the aberrant minority. Laws about homosexuality and abortion on demand are surely less important than laws that aim to set up good family-help policies that will create a healthier and happier society. It is the family that grapples with real life, that lives to the full and experiences the deepest emotional bonds. Education should stress the basic values of fidelity, mutual respect, understanding, and trust—qualities that can add dignity and a sense of responsibility to enrich the desirable freedom of this modern world.

2

Becoming a Mother

Even since I had my babies there has been a considerable change in the role of woman as mother and homemaker and there is no doubt that this is greatly confusing many women and their husbands even more. Let's have a look at the situation. Presumably you are several months pregnant and definitely going on with pregnancy or you would not be reading this book; but up to now you had choices that your grandmother did not have. You may have been using a contraceptive and chosen the time to have a baby, waiting until you had acquired a comfortable, reasonably secure way of living. You may even have "shacked up" for a while, under the mistaken impression that men can be tried out for size, quality, and color like a dress from a rack in a department store. You may even have got out of that situation by destroying a human fetus by abortion, believing that it was better to start again than bring an unwanted child into the world. (That it was un-wanted would have been denied by the many childless couples longing to adopt such a child.) You may have delayed marriage to become established in a career that grandmother could never have even contemplated. Maybe, like so many young people today, you both decided that engagement was commitment, but that it was convenient and less expensive to live with parents and not to have set up house until a child was on the way, when you both accepted marriage as necessary. This was risky and it robbed you of a lot of happiness, as well as depriving you of a valuable period of self-discipline and learning to understand each other. You may have decided to precipitate a decision in the shacking-up situation by becoming pregnant, because it is difficult to get a man to tie himself down when he is being fed and looked after and has his sexual needs met without any commitment to the future; so what else can a girl do if she really wants him? The trouble is that trapping a man rarely works for keeps. When grandmother's girl friends did it, society was on their side and the marriage was made to last. Now neither men nor women will go into a marriage by force unless one wants it desperately and the other has a troublesome conscience, and men particularly will not stay in a marriage that is not coming up to expectation. Rather strangely, too, men and women who have had many sexual adventures (please don't call them love affairs) before marriage seem to expect some magical change to occur in marriage that will enable them to fulfill each other's needs and desires without any further temptations or major problems in adjustment to each other.

You have probably worked at your job up to now and may be contemplating working up to the onset of labor—great-granny would have had the vapors at the mere idea. But can you cook and sew like granny and are there neatly piled towels and ironed sheets smelling sweetly of lavender in your linen cupboard and jars of preserves and homemade jam in your pantry? No, the supermarket jam is better than you can make and the ready-made clothes are easy to buy in a "disposable world." Frozen foods are readily available and you soon forget how much more delectable are the home grown. Great-granny could get a real sense of achievement from her domestic chores that modern urban woman cannot, and as she raised her ten children, only losing two, life was full. What time would she have had to do another job? And if great-grandfather did stray occasionally it was very discreetly and not far, and she had to close her eyes to it anyway, for she had given her life to her family. Lack of birth control methods had at times put a strain on the sexual relationship. Still, there was a security in her personal relationships; she knew what was expected of her and most of the time she was prepared to put her family first, caring for grandchildren, too, as they appeared. She was often overworked, at times resentful of man's freedom. Though she had demanded the right to vote and been given it, few of her sex served in Congress. She demanded education but was prepared to give the boys a better education than the girls. Father was head of his household.

But what of you, trained to earn a living, firmly intending to preserve your right to be a person and develop your talents as an individual, determined not just to be a housewife and not to overpopulate the earth? So far your marriage has been just for the two of you; you love each other, you even like each other. Although there are a few problems in sexual adjustment and in learning to put up with each other's habits, these are not insoluble. Now there is going to be someone else to consider, someone very demanding. You feel the trap closing in? Well, perhaps a little, but it is a delightful trap. You both want this baby.

What Matters Now?

Do you know what this baby wants from you? Do you know what really matters in life? This is a good time to think constructively about the kind of life you want. With a child reminding you of his presence with a punch or a kick and the extra weight to carry on your poor tired feet, let's see what matters most now.

Some material comforts, yes—that washing machine and fridge and a comfortable bed—but was that pale-fawn, long-haired, wall-to-wall carpet such a good idea, and what will a child do to that expensive living room suite and delicate wallpaper? Lucky you, if it's a rented house or an old one being done up as you go. Start on the kitchen and bathroom, but don't plan to have the carpenters in the week you come home from the hospital: Babies hate hammers.

Somehow the material goods are rather paling into insignificance beside personal relationships. Now you are really living, you are caught up in the future, the distant future that you will never see lies within you and you are afraid—not very fearful, but nothing means more to you now than a man who loves you, a reassuring arm around you, gentle, kind, reliable.

As Judith Wright puts it in her poem "Woman to Man,"

> *This is the maker and the made;*
> *This is the question and reply. . . .*
> *Oh hold me, for I am afraid.*

Now when you are needing protection and a time of peace to concentrate on rearing and nurturing your child you somehow face realities. Later you will be independent again, able to go back to your job if you want to, able to pay for someone to help you, able to build a barrier between yourself and the world again and toughen yourself; but now, while you are seeing a vision of the family you can have and the kind of marriage you want, why not talk about making it come true? Marriages that fail do so mainly because of failure of communication, failure to meet each other's needs through not knowing them rather than through deliberately not meeting them. They rarely fail primarily for sexual reasons, because it is not difficult to meet each other's sexual needs if you appreciate and love each other.

Your baby wants his own father and mother to rear him and he wants from you both much of what you want from each other—a warm, loving human relationship, kindness, understanding, interest, loyalty, truth and honesty, patience, excitement, new experiences, security and peaceful refuge when it's needed, encouragement and comfort when the going is hard. These are the things that matter in life. Most of them cannot be bought, and even those that can are better enjoyed with someone who can be trusted to consider what is in your best interest. Maybe that is what we want most: someone to consider our welfare while we consider theirs. Developing our interests and talents brings a sense of achievement and self-fulfillment—provided that we appreciate and encourage the interests and talents of our partner in marriage, accepting responsibility and giving freely of ourselves to create an environment in which a child will be surrounded by the things that really matter in marriage and in life.

Well, so much for the philosophizing. In plain English it means this is the time to take stock and see how well you are meeting your husband's needs before you decide he is not meeting yours. A wonderful thing about being pregnant and later breast-feeding a baby is that there is no question of priorities: The new human life has to come first. Even if it has you properly trapped, you have a wonderful excuse to look after yourself and expect father to put baby first, too; and of course, you have that time to think we've been talking about, a time of rest and reappraisal and renewal: not exactly R. and R. leave, but a very precious time that a woman needs. I really do feel sorry for the women who triumphantly tell me they came into labor at work and went straight to the hospital. Far too many of them come into labor tired and ill-prepared for the next few months, which are very important ones for themselves and the child and the establishment of the family as a family.

I am also sorry for the women who delay having a family for years after marriage, putting the emphasis on comfort and security. Babies greatly disrupt both, and the girl who has worked so hard to obtain them may find herself in quite a problem situation, assuming, of course, that she managed to become pregnant when she wanted to. The contraceptive pill is a common cause of infertility and an abortion can cause sterility.

Getting ready for a baby means a lot more than buying a crib and baby clothes and choosing a doctor and a hospital; it means looking at what being parents involves, and what a baby can expect as his rights, and the fact that he is not going to accept that you have any rights as parents.

I suppose it is because I am a pediatrician that I care so passionately about the welfare of children and believe that there is nothing more important for the future of the world than healthy, happy children. I do try to be scientific and factual, and I recognize that babies can be extraordinarily adaptable and grow well in a wide variety of family patterns; but I always come back to what father, mother, and child want most out of life, and I always end up with the need to care and be cared for, and to have a sense of the worthwhileness of what one is doing. This tremendous personal adventure of yours will involve you to the depth of your being. You are becoming a family. Dad is a very important part of it and needs to be involved in the preparations and to understand how his wife feels.

What Is a Good Mother?

If you are going to be a good mother, what is needed? Several studies, such as a famous one involving a thousand families at Newcastle-on-Tyne, have confirmed that the mother is of key importance. "In the study of these families and in attempting to correlate their environments with the health of the children, there emerged one dominating factor: the capacity of the mother. If she failed her children suffered. If she coped with life skillfully and pluckily, she was a safeguard to their health. In spite of lapses and failures, the mother stands out as the cornerstone of the family structure and our experience confirms that in all sections of the community she remains the chief guardian of child welfare."

There is nothing more certain than the fact that a mother can do a great deal to prevent ill health in her child and to promote good health. Health is emotional, social, and physical well-being, and it depends on three factors: heredity, environment, and the ability of the individual and society to manipulate the environment in which the individual lives. Unfortunately that environment is also being polluted and disturbed by factors out of our control, but the mother has a great deal of control over the environment of the baby both while it is in the uterus and for the next few years.

We have heard a great deal about the determinants of behavior from psychologists and sociologists and from observations on animal behavior and the effects of varying normal rearing patterns, nutrition, and other environmental factors. Anthropologists have studied tribal life and mother-child relationships in primitive communities and observed how mothers adapt their children to the environment and how they draw their needs and the children's from the environment. Some unfortunate experiments have been undertaken by well-meaning people who have tried to bring tribal people into civilized conditions too suddenly—in the name of equality, freedom, and the removal of racism—and thoroughly confused their cultural patterns. So there are now many sociologists trying to observe how primitive women rear their children successfully. It is always easier to study animals, because one can interfere with their environment with fewer pangs of conscience than with the environment of humans. The Harlow monkey experiments are the best known in this field. Harlow showed that female monkeys reared with artificial mothers made of wire, fur, and a bottle of milk could not develop normal maternal behavior to their young and had great difficulty even in forming a relationship with males for mating. Calhoun, working with overcrowded rats, showed that a female rat with no privacy and a passage through its cage failed to develop maternal instinct. I have met some Harlow monkey mothers and some Calhoun rat mothers who have been damaged by inadequate mothering themselves and cannot mother their young. Germaine Greer is a highly intelligent woman and in *The Female Eunuch* she recognizes that she would have trouble in mothering a child adequately and says she would like her child reared by a loving Italian family and would visit it for holidays. There is a terrifying passage in the British Council of Churches report, *Sex and Morality*, that sent a shiver down my spine, but is true: "A parent who is responsible for lack of love in the environment of a child sins against it as seriously as a stranger who assaults it in a park."

Women are not rats or monkeys; we have intelligence and the ability to have a good look at ourselves and our environment and our culture, and to plan; but these animal experiments can help us understand how we feel. Research shows that every pregnant woman has feelings for and against her pregnancy and also feels anxiety. So do not think you are unusual in that respect, and do not be afraid that you will not love the baby. But your feelings may be affected by the type of care you got as a baby and by what you expect of the baby, and even by his sex and your experience of babies. You will be given plenty of unsolicited advice during pregnancy and be regaled with many tales of other women's experiences. One woman will tell you what a delightful experience breast-feeding is and how you must not miss this experience; another will tell you how her nipples cracked and she hated the baby sucking and say that really you would do better not to try. One will tell you how the physiotherapy classes helped her and another that they were no help at all. One will say there is no need to let a baby interfere with your everyday activities or getting back to work—you can pay a good woman—and another tells you that the baby takes every minute of every day and she can't get the housework done or cook the meals. So much depends on the pattern you learned from your mother, on your ability to accept yourself as a woman and enjoy being a woman, on what kind of woman you want to be for your husband or yourself, and on what kind of homemaking skills you and your husband acquired before marriage.

Home Management

Unfortunately home management and everyday living are not examinable subjects at school, and until they are recognized academically, financially, and legally and have their place in college-entrance examinations that are equally applicable to men and women, homemaking will remain an unskilled occupation. However, you can learn a great deal during your pregnancy. There are good simple books on home management and nutrition, but it is more fun and you certainly learn more if you can join a course that has some practical work.

An understanding of nutrition is very important both for your diet during pregnancy and also in preparing food for your family, including the baby, later on. With inflation and rising food prices, the time seems to be fast approaching when we will not be able to have juicy steaks and eggs and bacon very often and will return to the much better balanced diet of less affluent countries. Most people do very well with half their calories from carbohydrate, one-quarter from protein, and one-quarter fat, so the basic national carbohydrates of Scotland, Italy, Asia, and Ireland (i.e., oats, spaghetti, rice, and potatoes) will compete with our sophisticated breads and breakfast cereals if we learn to cook them in an appetizing fashion with less expensive cuts of meat. It is much more fun selecting a diet and preparing food if you know the vitamin content of fruits and the food values of vegetables and how to conserve those values and still produce exciting meals. Just as the glossy magazines on making your house beautiful are said to have broken up many homes by encouraging expensive and too-frequent redecorating, many modern cookbooks make cooking far too elaborate and costly. In general, I find that men like their food straight and simple, unless they happen to be the kind who enjoy preparing it themselves; then they seem to make an overwhelming mess and use everything in the kitchen.

A study of children who were failing to thrive in the United States showed that less than half had a physical problem, 37 percent were not getting the right food in an acceptable way, and the rest either had emotionally disturbed mothers or were simply being neglected. In an affluent country where food was available, the mother's ignorance of food values and of a child's needs was causing malnutrition.

Prenatal Classes

Probably the most helpful information will be obtained from prenatal classes run by the hospitals or government health departments. The best type of course is a comprehensive one that includes preparation for childbirth and child care. It will consist of evening classes for both parents, usually four or five sessions, at which doctors interested in pregnancy and child care will give talks about labor, pregnancy, care of the young child, and the needs of mother and child, and perhaps there will also be an evening on man-woman relationships, the family, and family planning. There is usually a film and a demonstration of baby equipment, foods, layette, and also a question time. Having supervised such a course for many years, I am quite convinced that expectant parents find them very valuable, and even if the young moderns criticize the out-of-date films and kindly explain that modern educationists consider the lecture an old-fashioned method of communicating knowledge, the classes are packed to the doors, and until someone solves the problem of supplying highly qualified speakers in person and applying modern methods to large classes with voluntary lecturers this seems a reasonable compromise. There can even be a risk in using one modern method—group discussion. If the leader knows about groups but does not know the subject matter in enough depth, the discussions can be real pooled ignorance sessions. At least, at a lecture by an expert, the information should be correct and up-to-date, and someone is there to answer the questions. Even so, it may not be the information but the attitudes acquired that matter most. I remember asking one woman what she gained most and her answer was "an interested husband."

In addition to evening classes the hospital will also have physiotherapy classes that can assist you enormously in understanding labor, and the use of muscles, breathing control, and relaxation. Also, you may have some backache—most women do—and the change in your center of gravity puts strains on different places. Your new waddling gait may need some adjustment; the extra weight on feet that have been much abused in the past with changes in shoe fashion may produce some problems. The ligaments softened during pregnancy may welcome some physiotherapy advice, too. Most of all, the understanding of labor means you learn how to relax between uterine contractions in first stage, and how to use your energy most efficiently in the more tiring second stage.

The hospital physiotherapy courses are usually in the daytime, and working women may need to arrange to go to a private physiotherapist who gives classes in the evening. The hospital course is usually about six sessions, starting after the fifth month of pregnancy. At these pleasant social gatherings you get to know the others coming into the same hospital, chat over your minor problems and experiences, and ask the physiotherapist all those questions that you don't get time to ask the great obstetrician—in fact, quite a group-therapy session in a nice normal environment with a knowledgeable person in control.

There are also usually a couple of sessions conducted by the outpatient staff—a nurse and a physiotherapist—in which you will be taken to the labor room and shown how to use the anesthetic machine, where to go when you arrive, the charming hospital nightgown you will wear, and what an enema is. You also have an opportunity to meet some of the nursing staff and see the nurseries and generally get familiar with the setup. There will be a bathing and baby-care demonstration and a talk about preparing for breast-feeding, usually by a member of the nursing staff. This will all be done much more thoroughly in the hospital when you actually have the real thing to practice with, but it is a good idea to understand the general principles.

Statistics show that the main hazards a baby has to face can be greatly reduced by preventive measures. Prematurity is an associated factor in the deaths of half the babies that are stillborn or die in the first week, and the main causes of premature arrival are preventable, or at least they can be affected by prenatal care.

Toxemia, including kidney trouble and high blood pressure, hemorrhage, multiple births—all mean there is need for close observation. Coaxing the pregnancy on a couple of weeks more may mean a lot to the baby's welfare. A mother with a chronic illness, such as diabetes, needs very close supervision.

Labor and delivery of the baby used to present real problems, but it is now possible to estimate the size of the mother's pelvis early and the position of the baby, and most of the injury to the baby as the result of birth is now minor. A Caesarean section may be planned if real problems are expected. Of course some labors are still difficult, but hospital confinement has practically eliminated serious maternal dangers. It is a pity that the extreme sophistication of modern obstetrics is making some of the young moderns want to return to nature and have babies at home. That, however, is not returning to natural conditions: Even the most primitive tribes had people who were experienced in delivering babies, and they did not try to do it in a modern bed. Don't consider do-it-yourself obstetrics.

There may be other defects in your education that you could correct in the time before your child is born. You could, for instance, learn something about first aid, child care and child behavior, and dressmaking. To be able to give first aid is important. When junior falls off the fence or touches the iron or drinks a bottle of cough medicine, you will be the first on the scene, so to know some basic principles will ease your mind. Some knowledge of child behavior is best learned by seeing if a friend will let you bathe her baby and play with her children and baby-sit, provided they are not incubating measles or some other infection, at least in the first three months of your pregnancy. As for children's clothes, they are expensive and often almost designed to be grown out of quickly, so it is well worth acquiring some understanding of children's growth, an appreciation of the durability of materials, and enough dressmaking skill to make the simple clothes a young child needs.

Working During Pregnancy

In several countries now maternity leave is granted for six weeks before the birth of a baby and for six weeks after. Few doctors with the welfare of the baby at heart would regard that as ideal; but it is certainly better than nothing in a state where women are forced to work or where poverty is such that women have to work. Many pregnant women in light work will find that they can manage quite well until thirty-four weeks, but an office job that requires a lot of sitting will interfere with venous drainage of the legs and aggravate varicose veins and hemorrhoids. A job such as working in a store or nursing, where the woman will be on her feet a lot of the time, will have the same effect.

Professor Krupp, professor of gynecology and obstetrics at Tulane University, Louisiana, has proposed a plan for firms employing women who become pregnant. He says that they should stop work at twenty weeks, because pregnant women need rest: eight to ten hours at night and a rest period morning and afternoon with the feet up to take the pressure off the veins. He also says they should not carry weights or more than thirty-five pounds and should avoid chemically and physically hazardous jobs. Even he, however, having made good recommendations from the obstetrician's point of view, makes the mistake of putting the time before which no woman should return to work after the baby at only six weeks. I regard three months as the minimum, and that interferes with lactation.

The Art of Mothering

Margaret Ribble has defined the art of mothering as "to discover and satisfy the particular need of the individual child." Bearing a child does not make a woman a mother. She becomes a mother as she meets her child's needs. At first the way she meets his physical need for food, sleep, and elimination of waste is to him the measure and manifestation of love. These needs must be met appropriately or the world to him seems an unpleasant place. She provides the stimulation and she is the buffer that protects him from too much or unsuitable stimulation. Dr. Yarrow, comparing infant development with the extent of maternal care, found that the most important factors in the mothering were the amount of physical contact between mother and child, the child's environment, and the materials the mother provided that stimulated learning through his senses. A mother has to be sen-

sitive and adaptable and be able to accept her baby's individuality. She becomes involved to the depths of her being as
she accepts the protecting, nurturing role and gradually she
becomes a mother. Good mothers are not born, they are made,
partly by the example of their own mothers but also by learning
and preparing and discovering what babies need. So take
heart—this is living, and I have yet to meet the mother who does
not want to be a good mother. I know nervous mothers, mothers
running away from the job because of their lack of confidence in
their own ability, insensitive mothers, rigid mothers, unhappy in
their failure to be good mothers; but I have supreme faith in
women and their desire to do the best for their babies. This is the
time to learn and the time to get ready.

3

Father

Throughout history the father has been the provider and protector for his family. The ideal of manhood was characterized by physical strength, courage, and initiative, with a combination of common sense and intelligence perhaps better described as *nous;* the man found food and shelter for his family, and he fought the battles. The leaders in most societies were the men, old men of the tribe, founding fathers, men of wisdom, the decision-makers. No doubt their wives advised them at home, but ostensibly the man was the head of his household and the rulers were men. Society has changed; the needs of the family have not basically changed, but how they are met has. Where does the father stand now? What is masculinity?

Science can answer these questions with reasonable accuracy from research, but I always like to look to the artists: They are more sensitive than most of us to what is happening in the society they live in and I find they have much to say. Whenever I attend a medical conference in another city I like to wander around the art gallery. Mainly I look for pictures of mothers and babies, particularly breast-feeding, and there are a great many of these, tender, compassionate pictures with mother and baby totally absorbed. But I also look for pictures of children and families and everyday life. There are happy pictures of children at play, eating, sleeping, living. Looking for pictures of fathers painted over the centuries, I found innumerable paintings of strong, beautiful, vigorous young men; fighting men; hunters pitting their strength against animals, some horrifying in their hate and violence; sportsmen reveling in their skill; learned scholars; ascetics; sensitive men; mighty rulers; leaders of men; lovers, passionate, possessive, and caring; rapists, lustful and cruel; men teaching the young their trade and passing on their learning; men in every situation, expressing every emotion—but very seldom engaged in the everyday care of little children. Artists certainly see man procreating, fighting, protecting, teaching, reveling in physical prowess and just reveling—but not reveling in household chores or changing diapers.

A Mother Needs a Man

Sir James Spence says of being a successful mother: ". . . in this responsible task a woman needs a husband who will courteously and chivalrously provide shelter and protection and sustenance for her mind and spirit." What delightful old-world language! A woman may contribute a lot to the cost of the shelter these days, but protection and sustenance for her mind and spirit she certainly still needs. Women clearly need men to make the job of mothering easier, more fulfilling, and at times even tolerable. The father also has a more important job than ever in setting standards and limits and protecting his family from those who threaten the welfare of its members. This demands of him a new courage and wisdom and a greater awareness of his responsibilities not only to his own family but to the family of man in general, and not merely on a physical level but on an emotional and moral one—if we are to survive and have an earth to survive on.

Predators

Every animal and plant has its predators and there are several varieties: those that are parasitic, using and living on the host for their own gain; those that aim to destroy; and those that increase their own numbers and take over like weeds in a garden. In human society this third group are those who have been unable to conform to or accept the standards current in their society, and who, by recruiting people to their point of view, try to establish new standards. This is an acceptable technique for good or ill, an insidious and tolerated technique that can change the standards of a community by default of the majority. The rebels against the family and traditional moral codes are usually led by those who have failed in human relationships; they surround themselves by others who are different but have been unsuccessful in their own social group, and they try to make their own way of life appear attractive. I have often found that the enthusiastic female supporters of premarital and extramarital sex, the everything-is-all-right-as-long-as-you-use-a-contraceptive people, have had an abortion and/or a broken marriage. They have failed to find happiness, and sneering at and ridiculing the successful is an expression of their resentment.

The motives of the peddlers of pornography, the sexual deviants, and the anarchists should be crystal clear to all; but the ways of the believers in atheistic permissive philosophies (mainly spread by a few academics in the protected environment of universities) are more subtle. They wrap their story in jargon and sell the old line about freedom, self-expression, and sexual fulfillment to gullible young students who do not recognize all this apparently intellectual approach as a preliminary to seduction. These are people—both teachers and disciples—we hear agitating in the name of freedom for increased availability of drugs and pornography, and often assuming an air of worthiness and respectability by sponsoring such good causes as conservation and antipollution, and by nobly opposing war and oppression, usually at a safe distance from the danger and the work. They are rarely found giving their time or their money to the aged, the disabled, the destitute, or the disadvantaged. They disrupt meetings and lead protest rallies, but not protests against lowered standards in the community; in fact they are often at such protest meetings shouting down the speakers and doing their utmost to deprive others of their right of self-expression. Predators in search of personal acceptance, needing to justify their own behavior; predators selling their products through insidious, psychologically designed advertising; predators using mass media for their own ends to distort and conceal the views of others—and, most insidious and dangerous of all, predators in education interfering with the development of children. Excessive standardization and socialization of education make indoctrination of children to one particular philosophy possible.

These enemies of the family that I have been describing are the enemies of development of the individual within a free society. We need Parent Power, mature men and women alert to the dangers of modern society, if we are to combat them and show our children a happy fulfilling way to live at work and at play. It is father who must take the lead, and most women like their men to lead. It takes a mature adult to set limits to his own desires and recognize his responsibilities to the community; and it is the mature man who is most likely to find enjoyment and fulfillment in the lasting exclusive marriage relationship and the teamwork involved in rearing a family. There is no such thing as freedom without responsibility. And how can you be free if you are a slave to your own irresponsible desires and to the people who pander to them?

The Russian authority on the rearing of children, A. S. Makarenko, assisted by his wife, wrote a very interesting and enjoyable book on family life, *A Book for Parents*. In it he lays great stress on the father: "The care and upbringing of children is a big and terribly serious task and it is of course also a very difficult task. No easy tricks can help you out here. Once you have a child, it means that for many years you must give him all your powers of concentration, all your attention and all your strength of character. You must not only be a father and guardian to your children, you must also be the organizer of your own life, because your quality as an educator is entirely bound up with your activities as a citizen and your feelings as an individual."

Multiproblem Families

It is a well-documented phenomenon of Western society that the majority of social misfits and criminals come from a minority group in the community known as "the multiproblem families." In general they are low-income families, but their poverty is secondary to physical, emotional, intellectual, and moral poverty, poverty of spirit. They reproduce themselves by example through their rearing patterns, and they are the despair of the sociologists. The tender-hearted social worker, seeing their deprived state and not taught in her course how to succeed in spite of difficulties, often sees the answer in "radical redistribution of wealth" and "equal opportunity for all": admirable but useless if the recipients do not know how to use wealth or take advantage of opportunity.

Len Tierney, in *The Family in Australia,* reporting on a study of such families, observed that the reason for their poor social integration lay in the ineffective male who left the wife-mother to provide essential family life continuity, and in her failure to fulfill the dual role as she battled for the survival of her family. The husband-father, present irregularly and unreliably or absent altogether, never accepted responsibility and full involvement. The result was rearing of more males of low self-esteem, unsuccessful at school, incapable of satisfactory employment. They did not have adequate male models and leaned heavily on the peer group. They expected the female to carry the responsibility of the family. Tierney says, "It is suggested that the pivotal engagement of the multiproblem families with the wider society is found in the relationship of male members to work." If he is correct (and he produces strong evidence to support his hypothesis) educators and sociologists must face the challenge of strengthening the male sector of the community and defining the male role in modern society.

What Is Masculinity?

Is it solely by conditioning that boys become men, through the toys we give them and the behavior we expect of them? No observant, sensitive woman who has reared boys and girls from the breast to the university will ever believe that nonsense, though of course we do condition behavior or we would never establish the social patterns of living that hold the community together. What does the Y chromosome and the male sex hormone give to man that makes him different from woman? Strength, aggression, a leadership quality that makes him protect his family and gives him the kind of courage that is different from the courage of women; an ability to see the whole when a woman is taken up with detail and her emotional reactions; the active sexual role, the drive to insure the continuation of the race numerically but not the nurture of the young? Difficult, isn't it? Small wonder that subcultures are developing which try to eliminate sex-role sterotyping. But go to any man and woman who have lived and loved to the full and reared a family together and they will tell you that they accept each other as separate individuals with equal rights; they respect each other's integrity, individual interests, and need for self-expression and achievement; they meet each other's sexual needs; and their roles are complementary. There is a difference that pervades all they do, and they can only define it as sexual. Conditioned or inborn? Both, of course.

Hormones do matter. A boy's androgens increase as his testicles grow; his body changes shape; his muscle mass increases; he gets stronger; he reacts to sexual stimulation. In animals the injection of small amounts of hormones into the hypothalamus will produce mating and parental behavior. In tribal societies man had to use his strength and cultivate his aggression to stay alive and keep his family alive as he fought off enemies and brought home food; maybe the modern counterpart is that battle through the supermarket on Saturday morning carrying what his wife selects! In tribal communities Margaret Mead observed that men often carried babies and minded children while women gardened; but, she says, "No complex society with a written tradition has expected a man of stature and education to care for a baby." She does not see a basic drive toward the full fatherhood role such as women seem to have toward motherhood, but she does say that this interest men have in children in primitive communities may be a strong instinctive feeling in males to protect the young and helpless. Whatever it is, it is good and reviving, for men can rightly feel that this instinct is part of their masculinity. Fewer men now seem to say that children are women's work; but I do meet men who are confused about their father role, and perhaps a few of them are even male chauvinist pigs.

The mass media, particularly American TV shows, are apt to present the married man as a rather ridiculous, henpecked character at home, and an ogler of the female form away from home. Fathers are attractive only when widowed or divorced. These media also identify masculinity with sexual exploits, smoking, and alcohol. But I do not believe that most men care for the playboy image, or want to be seen as beings afraid of commitment and involvement, as escapists from reality.

Modifying of rigid sex roles is desirable; but it is sad to see that, in a New York study, children four to six years old from the unisex subculture did not know the difference between boys and girls.

Father's Importance to His Children

Many men see themselves—or, rather, think their wives and children see them—simply as a paycheck and a source of the weekly allowance, with the mother making all the real decisions. This is a very demoralizing situation, not improved by some of the more extreme women's libbers who seem to think that all they need man to be is a source of semen, and they can do the rest. I have heard a very competent female social worker say just that.

Fathers, take heart! There is an increasing volume of research that makes it quite clear that the father is very important indeed. He has profound significance in the development of the children, and most of all in their ability to accept their gender and their sex role in adjusting to society. Now is the time to take action to prevent your child from becoming a dropout, a delinquent, a homosexual, or a sexual extremist; you must become a real father to your child before he gets into his peer group.

Well, maybe that is being simplistic, but the signs cannot be ignored and perhaps I can elaborate.

There are studies of children's behavior correlated with father, with no father, and with an ineffective father. There are retrospective studies of delinquents' attitudes to parents, and of men and women in jail, and of their families. There is Sir James Spence's one-thousand-families study with ten- and twenty-year follow-ups; there is the ten-year follow-up of Dr. John Bowlby's work, *Maternal Care and the Growth of Love.* There are studies of men and women in their sexual relationships; and there is no doubt that father has a significant effect on his children's personality development that goes far beyond his contribution of half the hereditary characteristics and his emotional and physical support of the mother. After the first ten years the one-thousand-families study showed that mother was the keystone of her children's health and, as in Bowlby's book, made women more aware of their importance, even anxious not to fail their children. But the second ten-year follow-up showed that delinquency, marriage failure, failure to fit into society, failure to accept biological sex, either male or female, correlated with un-satisfactory or absent fathers. One study in a women's prison went so far as to say, "Women's prisons are after-care institutions for fatherless girls."

Fathers and Sons

There is much literature on father-son relationships stressing Freud's Oedipus-complex problems. Father is the masculine model for his son, the first man with whom he has contact, his hero, his yardstick for all men. Dad represents the outside world, so wonderful and exciting; dad shows him fire engines and takes him fishing; he knows all about everything, trains, airplanes, snails. Dad is big and hand-some and important to a little boy. Have you ever heard children boast about fathers at school? "My father drives a car like a racing driver"; "He has the most money"; "He catches the biggest fish." My little grandson's favorite expression is "me and my dad." Pity the poor child who has no father or uncle to boast about. No won-der he goes out and punches someone.

From father the boy learns how to behave to other people, par-ticularly to women. A study of American families and behavior of fathers showed that the men who helped their wives had fathers who helped their mothers. Father teaches him by his actions how to be a man and if he does not like what he sees he is in trouble with his sex role. He has problems with it, anyway; it is very hard to compete with this all-powerful wonderful hero as a rival for mother's love. Parents are often astonished at the violent reaction of a little boy when father kisses mother and a little figure suddenly dashes between them and pushes father away or kicks him. If father reacts aggressively, protecting his painful shin, he fails to understand the pain the green-eyed monster can cause, and he misses an opportunity of strengthening the family links by including the child in the family group.

Fathers often expect too much of their sons: They want courage, self-control, good table manners, and clean plates, long before a boy can give them. Father often demands this at a time when the boy is dealing with his complex emotional reactions to the bond between mother and father and may well feel like defying father and proving his independence with very disturbing results for family peace and sleep. The father who makes a friend of his son and shares the mother's love understandingly will remain a hero and even survive the devastating fall in prestige that occurs as children reach adolescence and see their parents as "square," or whatever the current term is by the time you read this book. Pedersen and Robson, in a study of American fathers and their children, also make an interesting observation that if fathers had a lot to do with their babies the boys responded earlier and more enthusiastically than the girls in greeting behavior. Margaret Mead suggests that it is important for the arousal of man's instinct to protect the young that he has early contact with the baby. So even the baby may eventually appreciate father's presence in the labor room!

Fathers and Daughters

No one really doubts that fathers are models, good or bad, for their sons, but what about girls? The evidence is that they are even more important for the girls. Again father has a head start on all other men. He is all men to his daughter and her image of him determines her attitude to men; the way he reacts to her in the first few years when she is just becoming aware of her feminine gender tells her what is acceptable feminine behavior. Research suggests that her father's expectation of her as a girl reinforces certain behavior and discourages other. If the father plays an active competent masculine role appreciated by his wife, then a girl grows up confident in her sexuality, socially better adjusted, and more confident in her other abilities. One study says that a father who "provides consistent discipline and is emotionally warm, stable and democratic, provides a highly significant ingredient to feminine development." So much for the "source of semen" theory!

There is evidence that homosexuality in males and females correlates more with unsatisfactory fathering than any aspect of mothering or other recorded data. Even if there is a genetic predisposition and hormonal factor suspected in some, homosexuality is environmentally determined.

Fisher, doing a detailed investigation of sexual response in women, also observed that a woman's ability to achieve orgasm in sexual intercourse with her husband was consistently linked with how dependable she had found those she loved and that her image of man as dependable was related to how dependable she found her father. "High orgasm" women saw their fathers as "men of high moral values and high expectations of their daughters" and "low orgasm" women tended to see their fathers as "casual, permissive, and short of definite values."

As Freud said long ago, mental health depends on good selection of grandparents; it has always been good advice to a young man courting to say, "Have a good look at her mother." Well, it may be more important to have a good look at her father. But don't despair. Just be more dependable and your woman will grow in confidence as a woman and more responsive to you, while you are developing the husband image for your daughter. If your daughter likes what she sees, she will choose a man of your values; if she does not, she may rush for comfort to the first male who apparently offers her "love" and she may be unable to distinguish "love" from the curiosity or excitement that often leads a boy to his first experience of intercourse. The father also influences the model his daughter has of women, because her mother is her first model and the way father meets his wife's needs and the responses he produces in her show the child the way a woman acts. If she is able to form a warm mother/daughter relationship, that also is important for her development as a mature, well-adjusted woman. Girls brought up without a father tended to show more aggression and more dependence on their mothers, more school maladjustment, excessive sexual interest, and social acting-out behavior. They also tended to despise men as socially and economically irresponsible, and these negative attitudes were passed on to them by mothers and grandmothers often involved in repeated unsatisfactory relationships with men. So the broken marriage tends to produce a broken marriage, and the illegitimate child reared with the mother tends to reproduce the pattern of extra-marital births.

Fathers and Mothers

Responsible, effective fathers can do a great deal for their children. Irresponsible, violent, and also excessively authoritarian fathers can do a great deal of harm. Huxley once wrote, "Give me good mothers and I shall make a better world." Lebovici, reviewing the literature on maternal deprivation and the effect of poor social conditions, changed this to, "Make me a better world and I shall give you good mothers." It could well be, "Give me good fathers and we will have better mothers."

This rearing of children is a family affair and a responsible male father figure is as important as a mother figure, not for mere survival but for coping with life. Father should be a stablizing force in his home; he relates his family to the outside world, though this is now being influenced by mothers going to work. Whereas mother used to have the final word about the home, food, child management, and father the final say about things outside the home, now mother is educated and has an active role in society and the duties and decisions are being shared more. Studies of Australian and American family patterns show that father is taking a more active part in the home and with his children. This in no way detracts from his masculinity. He gets to know his children better and to understand child development and behavior, so he is less authoritarian and more secure in his feelings about them. His opinion can carry weight and his wife and family can respect his judgment. If he understands them, he earns the gratitude of his tired wife as he backs her up in matters of setting limits on behavior and establishing guidelines, and the children can see how a good marriage works with its ups and downs and even get a glimpse of its ecstasy.

Father has an enormous advantage in one way over mother: He doesn't have to change diapers, put children to bed, bathe babies, or even read stories; but if he does, how much more everyone appreciates him! He can come in and be a great success as a father for an hour or so a day, and then he can go off to his nice peaceful job where law and order are respected. He can come home to chaos, firmly make a statement, and Johnny does at once what he has been refusing to do for the past hour. Father has much more opportunity for flexibility in his actions with children; mother has to maintain some kind of hour-to-hour consistency in management and routine that can be very trying for her.

The dual sex standard has now gone. To quote even Masters and Johnson, the sex experts, "The sexual climate in which children flourish best exists in homes where father and mother are comfortable with their own sexuality and their sexual relationship. Mother is happy that she is a woman and dad is even happier. Both are equally glad that he is a man."

When I wrote *Preparing for Motherhood*, I wanted to call it *Preparation for Parenthood*, but the publisher refused to allow it, saying that it sounded like a book on family planning. I still dedicated it to my husband and tried to stress the family, but it was not until I read Mavis Gunther's dedication of her book, *Breast Feeding*, that I saw put into words what I had wanted to say. She dedicated her book to her husband "who had great gentleness, strength and courage." Material gifts that a man has to offer, even Liz Taylor's diamonds, mean nothing compared with these.

4

Woman in Pregnancy

Your first suspicion that you are pregnant will come when you are "a few days late," but that is not always reliable. In these days of the contraceptive pill it is estimated that 30 percent of women have inaccurate or unreliable records of their menstrual periods. Ovulation is often delayed in onset after a woman comes off the pill, and some women have real problems in starting again. Emotional factors can also upset the dates. All the same, note the date when you expected a period; it can be very important in the last few weeks if the question arises of starting your labor early or doing a Caesarean section. There may also be a little bleeding at implantation of the ovum two weeks after conception, and this is not a period. Dates are also important if the doctor finds that the uterus is bigger than expected for the time. There may be twins or there are other reasons that he must consider.

The First Signs

If you begin to feel a little nauseated in the morning and your breasts are becoming more sensitive and fuller than usual, then the likelihood increases. Then one night nature calls you to the toilet from your warm and comfortable bed and you realize as you gaze at your sleeping husband that from now on children will make demands that only you can meet, and that your responsibilities have started in earnest. The enlarged uterus is pressing on the bladder, and this will irritate it, causing more frequent passing of urine until about three months. By then the uterus has risen up out of the pelvis and has room to stretch; you can sleep in peace again until near the end of pregnancy, when space is getting a bit cramped and there is again pressure on the bladder. Sleep in peace—that is, if the baby's kicking and some backache and perhaps cramps don't wake you.

The morning nausea usually lasts for a couple of hours and often disappears after three months; it is reduced by having something to eat before getting out of bed, so if your husband is not already trained to produce the early morning cup of tea then this is a good time to start. Sometimes the nausea lasts all day, sometimes it occurs only in the evening, and it is quite often associated with vomiting. It is always better to have some food in the stomach to vomit: Retching on an empty stomach is very unpleasant, as bitter yellow bile may come up. You may also find that you dislike some foods and crave others.

You will notice some changes in your breasts, enlargement and sometimes discomfort; and another hormonal effect is an increase in vaginal mucus and some discharge. If you are a smoker you may be fortunate enough to get a sudden aversion to cigarettes and be able to stop smoking suddenly. Nicotine crosses the placenta to the baby and does it no good; it constricts the blood vessels to the placenta and decreases the baby's food supplies, affecting his size, which may be approximately half a pound less at birth than the average. It also affects your heart and blood pressure and premature arrival of the baby. Smoking is simply not worth the risk, and if you have ever tried to give it up before you will realize the withdrawal symptoms that the baby may have to cope with when you withdraw his nicotine after birth.

As the first few weeks are such critical weeks for the development of the baby, don't panic and try to bring on a period; you may damage the baby. It is too early for the doctor to be sure that you are pregnant by examination until after you have missed a second period, but if you must know earlier then there are reliable pregnancy tests that can be positive as early as one week after a missed period and conclusive after ten days. The tests rely on the appearance in the urine of the hormone chorionic gonadotrophin, which is manufactured in the placenta. The first specimen of urine passed in the morning contains more hormone than any later one, so it is collected and examined in a laboratory. Testing used to be done by injecting the urine into mice or toads, but there are quicker antibody methods now available. You may even have seen advertisements in drugstores saying that pregnancy test kits can be purchased, but it is better to arrange for the test with your doctor.

Choosing a Doctor and a Hospital

The best time to visit the doctor will be a week after you have missed the second period. Now for the big decision—how to choose a doctor for this most important event of your life. Most women will visit the general practitioner to have the pregnancy confirmed and discuss with him the hospitals available and whether a specialist is desirable. Many general practitioners are very interested in obstetrics and have had a course of postgraduate training in an obstetric hospital. They are familiar with the local hospital and may also be more inclined to family-centered obstetrics and more personal service. All first babies should be born in a hospital with facilities for surgery and emergencies. You may well choose your hospital first and then find out which doctors are on the staff. Find out also if the hospital has a prenatal education program of classes for expectant parents and physiotherapy classes, and if possible whether the staff is interested in breast-feeding; a friend or neighbor may know more than the doctor about these classes, having once been on the receiving end. A hospital that trains medical students and nurses in obstetrics is certain to have a specialist staff, including anesthetists and children's specialists, and a high standard of obstetrical care. Many women find a woman obstetrician more understanding and approachable.

Having a baby these days is very safe for mothers because good prenatal supervision makes it possible to anticipate problems early and take preventive action, and to deliver the baby in a hospital with specialists available if necessary. It is essential to have a doctor you like and trust, because your obstetrician is going to become very important to you. Some women want a doctor who will answer all their questions, others are quite happy just to know they have a good doctor. The specialist obstetrician is also a gynecologist, qualified in all surgery of the female reproductive organs. Surgeons are men and women of action rather than words, and they are busy; you may find your visits short and be outside the door before your questions have been asked, so have them ready. The obstetrician works to a routine. There are observations he has to make every visit. His responsibility is to make sure that you and the baby are progressing normally and to see you through this experience safely and happily. He may be aware of all the worries most women have and answer them without being asked, but he may also assume that you are not worried if you don't ask. You are the customer if you pay the bill, and you are entitled to the service you want; but try to make it easy for the doctor.

The Medical Examination

The first visit will be the longest. You will have a full medical examination to make sure that your general health is satisfactory and your heart and lungs ready for the extra effort. Your height and weight will be recorded and compared with average height and weight.

Your weight will be checked every visit, since any sudden increase may indicate a problem in coping with fluid and salt and may be the first sign of toxemia of pregnancy. The doctor will give you an estimate of how much weight you can expect to gain. This is usually about twenty-four to twenty-seven pounds, and can be broken down as follows: baby, seven and a half pounds; breasts, one and a half pounds; uterus, two pounds; amniotic fluid, one and a half pounds; placenta, one pound; the rest is made up of extra fluid and fat put on by the mother. These measurements are approximate and will vary. Some women have babies that weigh up to ten pounds, with a correspondingly bigger placenta. Some doctors get a bit fanatical about weight, but excessive dieting is now definitely out of fashion and can be harmful both to the child and to the mother's ability to breast-feed. You can always cut down on refined sugar and white flour and have less fatty food, but no starvation days or fluid-only days such as you may have imposed in the past when you had only yourself to consider. In the latter part of pregnancy the weight gain is most significant, and one pound a week is about average; more than that might mean the fluid is collecting and blood pressure rising.

The blood pressure reading at the first visit is important for comparison with later readings taken every visit. The urine examination will show if there is any disturbance of kidney function; the doctor tests for sugar and protein, which should not be there; and if you have any frequency or pain on passing urine or have had kidney infections before, then he may suggest a fresh midstream specimen going to the pathologist for microscopic examination and a test to see if it has any organisms in it that could be causing infection. Bladder and even kidney infections are not uncommon in women. Protein in the urine is a sign of either kidney infection or toxemia. Eclampsia, the severe form of toxemia that causes fits, used to be very dangerous for both mother and baby but early diagnosis and the antenatal checks have almost removed it from the serious list, for it can be treated and controlled and if necessary the baby delivered early. Sugar may be passed normally at times even in 25 percent of women, but if it does occur the doctor will require a blood test to determine the level of sugar reached in the blood after a meal. A more detailed test may be required if the level is high, if there is a family history of diabetes, or if the mother is overweight or has had a very large baby before.

The doctor will do a pelvic examination by the vagina. This may be a little uncomfortable and you may feel embarrassed, but it is just one of those examinations you must get accustomed to and it is all in a day's work for the doctor, quite incidental and impersonal. He has to note the position and size of the uterus, compare it with the date of your last period, and see that everything is in place normally. He may also insert a metal speculum to enable him to see the cervix. This helps diagnose infection, enables a smear to be taken for culture and examination, and shows the doctor whether the cervix is holding tight and not getting too relaxed. Pelvic measurements are made to be sure that a normal-sized baby can get through the pelvis; if not, then preparations for a Caesarean section can be made.

The Tests

Once the doctor is satisfied that you are pregnant he will want a number of routine tests done. A chest X ray is advisable if you have not had one done in the previous six months, or at the most twelve months. This is to eliminate the possibility of tuberculosis, which still occurs and is particularly likely to spread in pregnancy. A sample of blood is collected from a vein for a number of tests. The hemoglobin figure shows whether the red cells have enough of the iron-containing pigment that carries oxygen around the body. Many women are anemic, and most need iron during pregnancy. Folic acid, which is essential for blood formation, is also frequently in low supply during pregnancy. The hemoglobin test may need to be repeated to be sure that the iron and folic acid are being absorbed if there has been some evidence of anemia; but the hemoglobin drops normally during pregnancy because of the extra fluid in circulation lowering the level—it is not a true drop, in other words; so don't get agitated if you happen to catch a glimpse of the figure on the report and see that it is lower than the first reading. The blood group is determined mainly to detect the RH-negative women, but also to find out what blood to use if you did need a transfusion, though that would be checked again and the blood cross-matched at the time. If you are Rh-negative your blood will also be checked for antibodies, that is, substances that have formed in the blood as a result of sensitization in a previous pregnancy that could destroy Rh-positive cells and could cross the placenta to an Rh-positive baby, causing anemia and other problems.

The sample of blood can also be examined for rubella (German measles) antibodies to find out whether you have actually had German measles before. If you have, and 80 percent of women have—many without knowing it, for the disease is difficult to diagnose and may occur very mildly—then there is one less worry. This also enables the doctor to repeat the test if you have any suspicious illness or contact with German measles; then if you have antibodies (and there were none before) the presence of the disease is proved and the question of termination of the pregnancy may arise. We know that the outlook for the babies in these cases is not as bad as we first thought, but there is a high risk of abnormality if German measles infection occurs in the first six weeks of the pregnancy.

Tests for syphilis and gonorrhea, the main venereal diseases, will also be done on the blood sample. Now, don't get uptight and insulted about this and refuse to pay the bill. Venereal disease has serious effects on the baby and can go completely unsuspected in women. In permissive societies venereal disease is increasing and becoming more difficult to treat. In the United States gonorrhea is commoner than measles and ranks with the common cold: Over two million people receive treatment in a year. Some doctors are no longer reporting cases, just treating the patient, and this means the contacts are not being followed up; so the more resistant organism is not responding very well to penicillin and people think they are cured. There is a very large pool of infection in untreated and undiagnosed cases.

Unfortunately people do not seem to realize that although contraceptives can prevent pregnancy and abortion can kill the unwanted embryo, neither prevents venereal disease. It can happen to almost anyone. I recently heard of a very respectable professor who had rather too much to drink at a party and woke up in a strange woman's bed. It is better to have hundreds of negative results than to miss one positive that could hurt the baby; so just feel grateful that your test was negative. Syphilis has increased and is more serious than gonorrhea for the baby because the baby becomes infected in the uterus, whereas with gonorrhea it becomes infected during labor. However, fortunately for babies, the increase in syphilis is mainly in homosexuals—though that muddled person, the bisexual, is dangerous.

Past Health and Previous Pregnancies

On the first visit the doctor will ask about past health and previous pregnancies. These are very relevant, so even if you have not confided in your husband about them you must, in the interests of the child, have no secrets from your doctor. Do not hide the fact that you have had an induced abortion. The British Perinatal Mortality study reported that a woman who has had an induced abortion must be regarded as presenting an increased risk and should have her baby delivered in a hospital. The reason for this is that the tightly closed cervix has to be dilated to allow removal of the embryo or fetus, and statistics show that in some cases this causes the cervix to open up spontaneously, causing miscarriage (particularly after three months) or premature labor with added risks to the baby. If you have had a previous baby the doctor will want to know about the labor, the size of the baby, and any complications; and he may want to write to your previous obstetrician.

He will examine your breasts, note nipple shape and size. Nipples develop with the breast increase during pregnancy so he will examine them again at about six months to see if any treatment is necessary and will discuss how you wish to feed the baby.

He will arrange future visits, probably monthly if all is well to about seven months, then twice a month, and finally weekly.

Danger Signs

There are certain danger signs that you will need to report promptly if they occur between visits.

Vaginal bleeding. This could be a miscarriage, but it may be from a polyp or an ulcer on the cervix, which can be treated; it could be due to the cervix beginning to open (incompetent cervix), and this could be tied shut. Any bleeding needs to be reported at once.

Abdominal pain that is severe or persistent. Cramping period pains are associated with miscarriage. If there is a backache and fever it may be pyelitis—that is, kidney infection—a fairly common condition during pregnancy and one that needs treatment.

Puffiness of face, eyes, hands, and fingers, marked reduction in amount of urine passed, sudden severe headaches, *blurred vision,* all suggest toxemia and need prompt attention. Swelling of the feet occurs with toxemia and should also be reported, but more often it is due to pressure on the veins and settles down overnight.

Changes in fetal movements. Babies do sleep and have quiet periods, but if movements become fewer than usual this could be significant.

Persistent vomiting can interfere with the fluid balance of the body and should be reported.

Normal Health

Most women look and feel well during pregnancy once the minor discomforts of the first three months are over, and "radiant motherhood" can become a reality. It is, however, very important to follow some commonsense measures for good health, and foolish to take risks. This means a nourishing, balanced diet, adequate rest, regular elimination of body wastes, regular exercise, good hygiene, and avoidance of strenuous dangerous exercise and of people with infections.

Family life is give and take all around—no martyrs! So father can adopt this healthy way of life for a while too, giving up smoking and keeping the alcohol to strict moderation, while mother sips her soft drink perhaps with only a little dash of something stronger.

Rules to Observe

FOOD

The diet has to provide all the baby's needs for growth, but that is not very much. A good sample for the day with all the basic needs would be:

Milk, about one and a half to two pints, or cheese, one to two ounces. These can be fat-free if you use cottage cheese or fat-free skimmed milk, which contain the calcium and protein.

Butter or polyunsaturated vegetable margarine at least one ounce.

Eggs, meat, fish, or poultry (protein): a serving of one of these two or three times a day. Liver or kidney once a week.

Fruit, two pieces, one being orange, tomato, or papaw, if possible.

Vegetables, potato and two others at main meal, salad if possible at another.

Cereal, a moderate helping, whole grain, e.g., a bran cereal or rolled oats. Bread, three slices of whole wheat.

The doctor may suggest a vitamin supplement and will almost certainly suggest extra iron and folic acid, and late in pregnancy you may have to reduce salt.

Keep the meals regular and simple: No long hours on your feet preparing fancy dishes that only increase your nausea with their delicious odors. Avoid fried food, pastry, and some of the leafy vegetables like cabbage if they cause indigestion.

REST AND EXERCISE

You will find that you are sleepy during pregnancy and glad of a daytime rest, so try to have an hour or so in the afternoon with your feet up to take the pressure off veins and the legs and pelvis. The traditional exercise has been the evening walk. Maybe the evening was chosen because granny was a little coy about appearance in pregnancy, or more probably she enjoyed the fresh air walk with her husband; now it may be very difficult to get him away from the TV. Housework is not sufficient exercise, tiring as it is; exercise in the fresh air and sunlight is much more suitable. In fact, if you normally play tennis or golf or swim, then keep on—but no playing to win anymore. Let that tricky ball go and never mind the long drive; you play for fun and relaxation now, and probably just swimming and walking are best in the later months. The keep-fit exercises are not approved by obstetricians; much better to join the physiotherapy class and learn the exercises that relieve backache, and learn how to relax as well as contract muscles.

HYGIENE

Showers are preferable to baths; at least do not soak in hot baths. Hair may be washed as usual once a week in spite of old wives' tales. Hair is apt to become dull and come out and also to darken, but don't worry about this; after baby arrives it thickens and grows again, maybe a shade or so darker. Who worries about color these days, when your best friend suddenly turns up as ash blond or even gray, and granny has gone blue?

Your complexion may suffer, even though it may be clear of pimples and look very healthy; many women, particularly brunettes, develop the mask of pregnancy, a darkening of the skin across the nose and cheeks, a dark line on the tummy, and marked pigmentation around the nipples. This is all due to action of the adrenal gland and is quite normal and fades after the baby arrives. Use a powder base and cover up the telltale mask.

TEETH

There is an old wives' tale that says every baby costs a tooth, but there is no need to let that happen. Baby certainly has first claim on the calcium, and if the mother's diet is deficient in milk or a milk substitute then her teeth may decay more. Teeth should be cleaned regularly with a medium or soft brush, perhaps even with a toothpick, since gums are often tender and swollen and liable to bleed. Your dentist may recommend a tooth powder and some extra vitamin C. Dental work needed is usually done between the third and seventh month when X rays and local anesthetic are safer. If you live in a fluoride-deficient area, then a fluoride tablet a day will help you and the baby.

BOWELS

Constipation is a common problem during pregnancy and greatly aggravates hemorrhoids (piles). The uterus is growing and pressing on the bowel, so the movements should be kept soft and strong laxatives avoided. It is best to eat extra roughage, e.g., whole grain cereal (particularly bran), fruit both fresh and dried (prunes, figs, raisins), and to drink extra fluid, even just water. Above all, answer the calls of nature promptly; don't leave a movement to accumulate in the bowel and press on the sluggish veins. If you do need a laxative make it a mild vegetable one, more a softener, like those derived from senna, figs, or prunes.

CLOTHES

I never cease to be amazed at what some women wear when they are pregnant. Somehow fashion's latest atrocities become magnified. When I was in the United States I went to a prenatal evening for women in the later months of pregnancy to hear a talk on breast-feeding. I saw women in hot pants, bare midriffs, jeans, every color of the rainbow, scarlet being not at all unusual.

Maybe militant motherhood is the message in a country with such a poor marriage record, but it took me days to recover from what the friend who took me called my "cultural shock."

Perhaps I should just give you a few general principles. You will not feel the cold, so don't plan for close-fitting woolens. You will hate anthing tight and constricting around your body and legs. You will often feel a bit blown up with indigestion, so loose waists and clothing hanging from the shoulders are the most comfortable. Allow for your bust measurement to increase up to four inches, at least two, and your hips not very much. You sweat more than usual, so easily washed clothes and white collars feel fresh and good for the morale. Clothes are great morale boosters. Underwear is comfortable and attractive these days, washable, no bones, and gently supporting. The main considerations are to avoid direct pressure on the baby, support the lower part of the abdomen, particularly for second and later babies, and avoid constriction around the waist and thighs that will press on veins. For a first baby the muscles are firm and you may not need any support until the fifth or sixth month when you will be ready to get both your feeding brassieres and a panty girdle with no legs or short ones.

Discomforts and Warnings

There are a few common discomforts that perhaps a few words of advice may help to reduce.

CRAMPS

Leg cramps are very common, particularly after a long day on your feet. The pain is quite agonizing and due to muscles contracting and not relaxing. Rubbing or walking about will help, but a hot-water bottle to the spot is quickest. A good pinch of salt and a drink may act like magic but may not be permitted on the diet. Too much milk is suspected as an aggravating factor. The pain of cramps is something one does not suffer in silence and quick relief is essential; and here husbands really are invaluable, for filling hot-water bags, rubbing sore spots, and enveloping you in comforting arms. In moments like these you will really appreciate your double bed. Don't let any poor deluded unloved modern talk you into twin beds at any stage of your married sex life. It is very reassuring and pleasant to find welcoming arms and a warm bed when you come back from those nocturnal trips to the toilet or to the kitchen for a snack. Sleep may be elusive and fear may stalk in the night, and there is nothing like a nice warm husband to remove one's anxieties.

INDIGESTION

Most pregnant women have some digestive upsets: nausea, heartburn, vomiting, pain after meals, wind. If you have not been able to get father to cooperate over that early morning cup of tea, then a thermos of hot tea or a glass of lemonade will work as well. There has been a great deal of nonsense talked about vomiting in pregnancy, but most women who vomit are not emotionally disturbed and they do want their babies. Occasionally one sees a severe vomiter who is having problems adjusting to her female role and accepting motherhood, but there are also probably hormonal causes for even severe vomiting. I know women who vomit with their daughters and not their sons and vice versa. Some mild sedation may help, but make sure a doctor prescribes it.

HEARTBURN

This is a very common complaint, affecting about two-thirds of all pregnant women. It is a kind of indigestion, a warm feeling of discomfort in the pit of the stomach and behind the breastbone, aggravated by food and changes of position. It appears to be caused by the relaxing of the sphincter around the base of the esophagus (the entrance to the stomach), which allows the acid contents of the stomach to come up into the esophagus and irritate it. The relaxation of the sphincter can be caused by hormones (probably increased during pregnancy) and also by smoking. A few practical suggestions for relieving it are: having small meals and avoiding large ones; drinking milk and alkaline mixture as necessary; avoiding bending and lying flat; and, if you are obese, losing weight. Smoking must be given up.

CHRONIC ILLNESS

If you have any chronic illness, such as diabetes, kidney trouble, heart disease, tuberculosis, epilepsy, or problems with past pregnancies, then you may also need a specialist physician to examine you and keep an eye on your treatment. Medicine is very specialized these days. Changes may even have to be made in regular medication, so discuss this with the doctor. Report any symptoms and do not attempt to treat yourself, because so many medicines cross the placenta to the baby.

STRETCH MARKS

These appear on the breasts, thighs, and abdomen, and depend on how elastic your skin is. They can look very unsightly and red, but they will fade later, and rubbing with oil may help.

VARICOSE VEINS

Blood in the veins of the legs flows up from the toes on its way back to the heart. The veins contain valves that help this process. During pregnancy the vein walls are relaxed by a relaxing hormone and there is pressure from above from the enlarging uterus, so the veins may become dilated. Since blood is also sent back to the heart by muscle movement in the legs, the prevention of varicose veins can be helped by exercise, e.g., walking or wriggling toes and bending legs. It also helps to have a number of short rests during the day, to get the feet up above the body and lessen the pressure, and if necessary to wear supporting panty hose.

Emotional Aspects of Pregnancy

These days every woman's magazine runs supplements on What You Should Know about Pregnancy, Questions the Pregnant Woman Asks, and What Every Girl Should Know about Conception, Birth, and Contraception. If you don't know the physical facts you have been closing your eyes or mind to them, or maybe you only read what is relevant to you at the time. The physical facts don't vary much from magazine to magazine, but what about the emotional and the social aspects? You read all those woebegone letters about the baby blues and the loneliness, and you know that mental illness is the commonest health problem of our modern civilization, and you wonder if you really want to be a mother at all. Well, every woman goes through quite an emotional upheaval during pregnancy and in adjusting to the arrival of the baby, and it is quite normal to feel anxious. Recently, I read an article in an obstetrical journal indicating that the women who had nightmares and worrying dreams before the baby arrived often had the best labor. So let's have a look at what normally happens.

Bearing a child is the greatest creative act a woman can perform. It has been called the fulfillment of every woman's most powerful wish, a time of becoming a mature person, a period of growth into womanhood. As in infancy, entry into adolescence, and menopause, there is a kind of reappraisal of oneself and finding of oneself. What kind of person am I? Can I do this task ahead? Wouldn't I rather run away? I don't want to fail my husband and let my mother down. Childhood is past, the freedom of adolescence is past, even being one person is past, and acceptance of a new life developing within one's body is the first emotional hazard to deal with. The first three or four months produce some very mixed feelings. Even women who have wanted a baby very much may begin to wonder if they still do, and to be fearful about themselves. They feel very tired, at times a little faint, nauseated, and vomiting, and not very happy about this joyful event. Having now proved your fertility and your husband his virility, that worry is over; but are you now ready to be father and mother?

At this time some women seriously contemplate abortion and feel very guilty about their mixed-up feelings. All kinds of emotions from the past are stirred up, particularly for those who have had an abortion or come from unhappy families with poor examples of home life. Then there is the granny-to-be, your mother: She may reject the idea of becoming a granny, she may worry about your health and safety, or she may think it all wonderful and want to take over—and she may even be jealous. Anyway, this means a new, changed relationship with your mother, usually a better understanding between you. Proving yourself a woman in your adolescent years usually meant a few storms, but now with a husband and your baby on the way you and your mother can find a new mother-daughter relationship as friends, and you can look to your mother to provide experience and support through this new adventure. Your husband can be with you through the labor and be a tremendous support, but your mother *knows,* and somehow this does break down some quite considerable barriers. Girls who have not had the experience of good mothering themselves often have fears that they cannot love and care for a baby. They begin to feel uncertain even about their marriage, and may be disappointed and depressed and fearful. You have read that people from broken marriages tend to have broken marriages and that unloved children tend to grow up into unloving adults; but forewarned is forearmed. Love, concern for the well-being of another, is a very powerful force indeed, and even if your pattern has not been good, love is something one learns. Sir James Spence, a very great pediatrician, said that every mother must fall in love with her baby, and that love relationship usually begins seriously when it begins to move within you and you become really aware of the growing child. The unpleasant symptoms of the first three months will disappear, and you begin to see yourself more seriously as a mother and to feel good about it.

The women who ignore the existence of a baby until the world can see that it is on the way are often shutting out reality; and in those who accept the reality a few worries and fears are quite in order. Psychotic illness is rare, but anxiety is common and it is not hard to deal with; so talk about it either to your doctor or to a friend who has a young baby.

Most women as they get into the last three months feel more helpless and dependent on others, have less desire to be active, and can in fact feel very irritated by their sense of dependence when they have been very active independent people. But this is normal too, probably part of nature's plan to make you rest a bit more and orient yourself in the new role. It is quite normal to be concerned about labor and the welfare of the baby, and here is where preparation-for-childbirth classes can be a real help and reassure you about many of the fears you do not like to express to your doctor. Every woman wonders what her child will be like and fears that he may have some abnormality. She may also fear for her own life. Her doctor will reassure her, but nothing can remove occasional irrational fear. Childbirth is part of normal life for most women, and the best insurance you can take out against things going wrong is to find a good doctor and visit him regularly; rest, get plenty of exercise, and follow a sensible diet; and don't dwell on those fears. Fear, anxiety, and fatigue can affect labor; knowledge and preparation can reduce fear. From the moment you become pregnant you are part of another person's future. Your peace of mind, your happiness, your diet, your general health—all influence the baby. And you should expect a little special attention: comforting arms to soothe your fears at night, gentle but just as satisfying sexual enjoyment, and more consideration for your needs. Do allow yourself some time at home before the baby arrives, and don't go into labor tired and emotionally unprepared for the baby. A woman who does this is often soon back to work. She must artifically feed her baby and leave her baby to someone else—a kind of rejection of the maternal role and of the child. If you are forced back to work by financial necessity or tempted back by maternity-leave policies, then find alternate ways of expressing your maternal love: time baby's bath, naps, and meals so that you can be there for most of them. Long hours of separation in the early months make it more difficult to establish the bonding so necessary for a good mother-child relationship. A good start makes for good relationships throughout life. The path through birth, infancy, school years, and adolescence is not smooth, and the foundations for loving, supporting, guiding relationships as well as for constant conflict are laid down in the early years. Enjoy and understand them!

5

The Unseen Child

Every woman who has borne a child has dreamed of what that child is like as it slowly grows inside her body. At least from the first uncertain fluttering movements that she felt, it became a person, more real than in the first few months when he mainly made his presence felt for his mother through her nocturnal trips to the toilet and her distinct aversion to food. Those movements, described by the more romantic as like butterflies' wings and by the more prosaic as like wind in the bowel, are really quite a late sign of the baby's presence. The woman having her first baby will probably not recognize them until she is twenty weeks pregnant, but next time it is easier and she will be fairly sure by sixteen weeks. Actually, the baby started moving his arms and legs at about eight weeks, but they were so tiny then that the ripples they caused in the amniotic fluid were far too small for her to detect. But let's go back to when it all began, this human life that your love created!

Fertilization

Two weeks before the menstrual period was due Nature had an ovum ready. Follicle-stimulating hormone (FSH) from the pituitary gland had ripened it and luteinizing hormone (LH) caused it to be released into the abdominal cavity where the waving tendrils on the end of the Fallopian tube, rather like an anemone, lured it into the tube with firm insistence. There it met the sperm, sometimes described as like trout swimming upstream, their tails propelling them along, the big ones carrying X chromosomes to make girls and the little ones Y chromosomes to make boys. It seems that the little ones move faster, and it is suggested that the nearer intercourse occurs to ovulation the better the chance of having a boy, because one of the millions of the small, more agile Y chromosome sperm gets to the ovum first. In fact, the baby planners quite seriously advise that if you want a girl it may be wiser to have intercourse a day or so before ovulation, because the Ys get there too soon and don't live as long, and the Xs arrive at the right time; it is also suggested that a little manipulation of the acidity of the vagina by douche or vaginal pessary may make the environment more agreeable for the sperm of your choice. So though it is the father who determines the sex of the child, since he alone has the Y chromosomes and a boy needs XY and a girl XX, it seems that mother may have some power of selection. Perhaps you can't blame father for those five delightful daughters and those expensive wedding receptions you see in the future.

Chromosomes and Genes

In the Fallopian tube the sperm and ovum unite to form a new individual human life. Though the ovum is smaller than a decimal point and the sperm or spermatozoon (to be more technical) is infinitesimal, together they contain all the genetic material needed to grow into a child. Both sperm and ovum were carrying half the necessary chromosomes—that is twenty-three each—when they met, so together they made up the twenty-three pairs that constitute the human quota. We know now that every cell of the human body contains these forty-six chromosomes, and on each chromosome in a definite order are hundreds of the genes that carry our hereditary characteristics. These genes are in pairs along the chromosome; each member of a pair represents the same characteristic—the color of the eyes, the shape of the nose, for instance—but one will be likely to be dominant and show up, while the other remains hidden or recessive until in a later generation it meets another of its kind. These genes consist of deoxyribonucleic acid (DNA) and ribonucleic acid (RNA), the basic stuff that life is made of; DNA is the double helix that won its discoverers a Nobel prize. When Nature was preparing the sperm and ovum for their great moment, she split the chromosomes down the middle longitudinally, separating the gene pairs and reducing their number to twenty-three, so when the chromosomes from sperm and ovum united with each other a new gene pair was formed. Geneticists are very near to cracking the genetic code and mapping the genes along the chromosome so that sometime in the future they may be able to detect the genes carrying hereditary diseases and perhaps treat or remove them.

In the meantime your baby, with his own unique arrangement of genes, is on the way. Maybe you two brown-eyed, dark-haired people were each carrying a recessive blue-eye and a recessive fair-hair gene and that was the one you both passed over. If you find yourselves with a blue-eyed blond the hospital staff will not have given you the wrong baby—it will just be that recessive characteristics were passed on; but it is three times more likely that the baby will be brown-eyed and dark-haired. Though each gene carries a particular characteristic, genes do have what we call different penetrance, and offspring do not necessarily turn out just like fathers or mothers but may be mixtures of both heredities. Moreover, several genes may influence each other, so it can need two or three together to produce other characteristics. Even then we talk of some conditions as being genetically predisposed and environmentally determined: Conditions like some mental illnesses, such as schizophrenia and depression, may be commoner in some families but less likely to occur in the stable, loving family even if the gene has been passed on. Studies of uniovular (identical) twins, that is, twins from the same ovum, are helping unravel these mysteries. There are situations in which the twins have been separated and reared in different environments and yet still look identical; but they can have IQs differing as much as fifteen points, showing that certain basic intelligence is inherited but that environment can develop it. The genes can also be affected by some viruses and drugs and not turn out quite the way nature intended.

Implantation

Whatever you may think of that ultramicroscopic particle hurtling down the Fallopian tube—or perhaps I should say rolling gently down for about three days—to implant in the wall of the uterus in a few days' time, the die has been cast, and nature has decreed what the child will look like, and what will be his basic talents, whether he will be tall or short or sensitive or tough, whether musical or tone-deaf, whether a potential Olympic swimmer or a potential Dr. Schweitzer. The cells of the fertilized ovum divide and subdivide quickly within a few hours of fertilization until they soon look rather like a raspberry through the electron microscope; and the cells are nourished by the tiny yolk. In the meantime the hormones from the pituitary, the

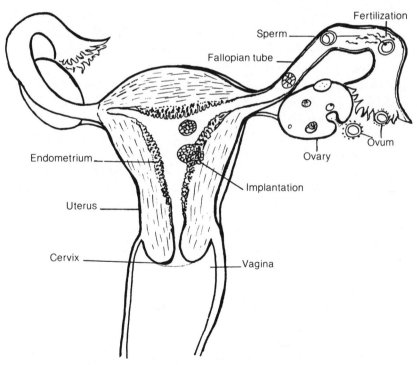

Pregnancy: ovum to implantation

gonadotrophins, are stimulating the production of progesterone and getting the wall of the uterus thickened and ready for the little ball of cells to implant and dig in and form itself a comfortable spot in which to develop. Now the developing ovum produces its own hormone, chorionic gonadotrophin, and this keeps up the production of estrogen and progesterone and controls the lining wall of the uterus to assist in the implanting process. It also acts on other parts of the mother's body to prepare her for nurturing and bearing the child; her breasts feel fuller and her nipples more sensitive. Implantation finishes the ovular phase of development, and the ovum now becomes an embryo and the recognizable human characteristics start to develop.

The Embryo

They say man climbs up his evolutionary tree in the first twelve weeks, and that seems to be what he does do as each organ of the body goes through stages of development that finally end up after twelve weeks in the final form. From then on, it is mainly growth and more sophisticated development. Let's have a look at this fascinating development when, as the old psalmist says, "Thou didst knit me together in my mother's womb. Thou didst fashion my inward parts."

During this early phase the little ball of cells formed itself into a hollow sphere, the blastocyst, with a collection of cells in one part that we call the inner cell mass, which will develop into the baby. The other cells of the blastocyst form the trophoblast, and this has a special power of burrowing in and embedding the blastocyst: It puts out fingers of tissue that reach into the lining wall of the uterus and make cavities through which maternal blood circulates and brings food and oxygen to the embryo. This occurs about the time the mother's menstrual period would be due, and the implantation may result in a little bleeding, but not nearly as much as at a normal period.

The trophoblast has usually chosen a site high up in the uterus near where the blastocyst entered from the Fallopian tube, and this area now rapidly develops into a complex system for feeding the baby, removing waste, and producing hormones; and it becomes known as the placenta (you may see it as the afterbirth if you really want to, but it is not a very pretty object). It eventually weighs between one and two pounds and is about the size of a dessert plate and approximately two inches thick in the middle. Sometimes the blastocyst falls too far down into the uterus before implanting and the placenta may form low down near the neck of the womb or even across it. This does not interfere with the baby's development, but it is an awful nuisance when the baby wants to get out at birth, and a Caesarean section may be required; also it may cause bleeding.

The first change that occurs in the inner cell mass is differentiation into three layers of tissue: first the ectoderm, which is the tissue from which the skin, hair, nails, brain, and nerves develop, then the endoderm and the mesoderm. The endoderm forms all the digestive system and the lungs and some of the glands; the mesoderm forms the muscles and lining tissues. It is fascinating to think that every animal on earth develops in this way, with three layers that develop into the same parts of the body; and even at this primitive stage that tissue knows whether it is to be the golden hair of a little girl or the scales of a fish.

The ectodermal tissue forms the neural tube and crest in the third week. This is to be the brain and nerves, and, as the most important part, no doubt it forms first. In a few days the primitive heart begins to form. At first it is just a collection of blood cells in a cavity, then the cavity wall thickens, its muscle starts to pulsate, and in six weeks we have a one-cavity tubular heart that can pump blood along to the placenta to pick up the baby's needs. It twists and turns upon itself and forms into four chambers that connect with each other. The system that will be needed to take blood to the lungs for oxygen when the baby is born is developed now, but since it is not needed in the uterus there is an amazing system for allowing only some blood to pass to the lungs to make sure the passages are kept open while the rest is brought from the placenta along the umbilical vessels straight to the heart of the baby. The brain has first priority for oxygenated blood, then the other tissues get their share.

It is a convention to measure the duration of pregnancy from the first day of the last period ("menstrual age"), but really the first two weeks of that time the ovum is only developing and not fertilized. So you may be a bit confused when the doctor says you are eight weeks or twenty weeks pregnant, and think that this does not fit what I am saying. Well, being a pediatrician and knowing that the baby started at conception, I like to talk of the "fertilization age" or the age from within a day or so of ovulation.

At four weeks the embryo is about one-fourth of an inch long and weighs about a thousandth of an ounce. The brain, being the most important organ, is a prominent bulge at one end; the spinal cord, with the vertebrae and muscles, is discernible down the back, ending in a very distinct tail that will disappear later; the heart, at this stage, is an S-shaped tube—it started pulsating at twenty-five days; the tube of the digestive tract is beginning to twist and elongate and has just burst out at the top to form a mouth. With a microscope, the beginnings of liver, intestinal glands, thyroid, gall bladder, pancreas, and lung can all be distinguished. The embryo is beginning to look like some kind of animal; eyes and ears are there, and there is a semblance of a face. Changes occur daily that soon reveal the human form that has been there from conception.

By six weeks the eyes have moved around to the front. Projections of tissue growing around from the side of the head and neck meet in the middle to form the palate and the lower jaw, and meet tissue growing down from the front to form the nose; this is regarded as the fishy stage of development, as the evolutionary gill slits of fish are visible as the neck projections meet and fuse. It is at this time that, very rarely, abnormalities such as harelip and cleft palate occur through faulty contact of the growing ends, but these days surgeons perform miracles of plastic surgery that make any abnormality hard to detect. The heart and liver are now clearly recognizable and on each side of the embryo there are buds of tissue protruding, rather like little flippers but rapidly forming fingers and toes; so the limb buds become arms and legs. The embryo is growing very fast and every cell is important, so that if anything happens to disturb its growth a serious abnormality can develop. A poison like thalidomide, on the critical day of development, can stop the limb buds growing; the virus of German measles infecting the embryo may damage heart, brain and eyes. The embryo is now about half an inch long. The skeleton is forming in cartilage, the stomach and intestines are moving into their final places in the abdomen, and the pituitary gland is forming.

By eight weeks there is no doubt whatever that this is a human being. His eyes and ears and nose are now a face; he has fingers and toes; he has a fat little tummy full of liver and gut, but it does not all fit in yet, so quite a large hernia still projects into the umbilical cord; he is about an inch and a quarter long; the soft cartilaginous skeleton is now calcifying to form bone; the heart is fully formed and beating in the same way as the adult heart, but much faster; his cardiogram can be recorded, and is very much like his dad's. The sexual organs are developing, too, but Nature does a strange thing: She prepares for male and female with two

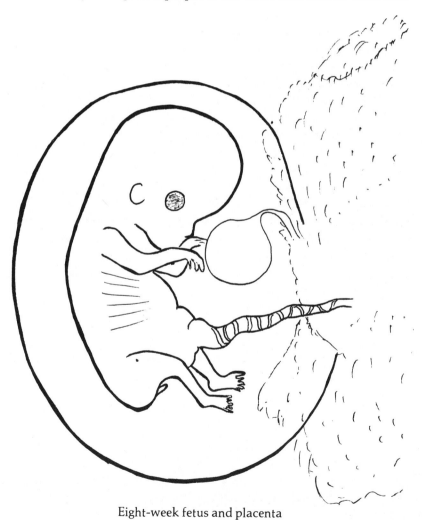

Eight-week fetus and placenta

sets of sex equipment. This is the only time in life when male and female can be the same; after this point the parts not needed will degenerate and a male or female will emerge. Nature has no patience with unisex, but now and again some mix-up happens and both male and female organs develop together, or part of one and part of the other.

The Developing Fetus

It is in the development of the kidney that the baby seems most obviously to climb the evolutionary tree, because nature forms three different kidneys one after the other. The first is a simple one that does not excrete waste to the outside of the body. It is called the pronephros, as is the kidney of some very simple fish; then it forms the mesonephros, which works more efficiently; but very soon that disappears too, and the final metanephros that will develop into the adult kidney forms. It excretes urine into the amniotic fluid. The amniotic fluid is the fluid contained in the membranes surrounding the baby, the bag of waters you will hear about when labor comes; in fact it may start to leak somewhat inconveniently when labor starts.

This amniotic fluid is a cushion, a water bed, that protects the baby and it also enables the baby to practice some of the body functions that it will need to perform alone when it is born. In the uterus the baby swallows amniotic fluid: it passes through the body, and water and protein are absorbed, and some is passed out by the kidneys as fluid back into the amniotic fluid again. This sounds like a somewhat unhygienic arrangement, but don't worry: The waste products are collected, taken to the placenta, crossed to the mother's bloodstream, and disposed of by her. Baby does not normally have his bowels open before birth and the amniotic fluid is quite sterile. The waste is more safely and more efficiently processed than the recycled water from our sewage treatment plants, and no strikes or industrial troubles either!

Well, here we are at twelve weeks, all organs present and correct, in the right place and functioning, even if in a very elementary fashion for some organs. The fetus is three inches long at this time, and although he weighs just under an ounce, his proportionately big head makes him too heavy; he is swimming around, arms and legs moving, fingers and toes curling; he can make a fist and frown, he makes sucking movements; though the eyelids are still sealed tight, he squints his eyes; breathing movements can now be demonstrated, though it is amniotic fluid that goes in and out of the lungs. Study of this fluid shows that now the hundreds of thousands of tiny filters in the kidney are beginning to work. Twenty little tooth germs have started to form in the jaws; bile is passing into the intestine from the liver and the bile pigments will accumulate and give their dark color to the first bowel movements; the sex organs are now quite distinct, and the external genitals quite definitely male or female, though the testes are still inside the abdominal cavity. The heart has been estimated to pump close to fifty pints per day around the body and to the placenta. There will still be some refinements of hearing and sight to develop, and the brain will become more complicated; but the electroencephalogram shows brain waves, and the electrocardiogram shows heartbeats and electrical impulses.

I recently had the soul-searching experience of serving on a church committee to collect information that would inform the church and assist the theologians in their thoughts about abortion, and here I found people who did not believe that this twelve-week-old fetus was a human being. They granted that it was biologically human, but would not admit that it had a soul or was a person or could "think." My embryology teachers had unfortunately omitted to educate me on the embryology of the soul and no recent books had any reference to it; so I was inclined to play safe and decided that if the Creator had everything else in place by twelve weeks then it was not for me to say the soul was missing, and that if the electroencephalogram showed brain activity who was I to say the fetus could not think in some primitive fashion? The real issue, of course, was whether it was quite all right to destroy the developing child at the whim of the mother, or whether she had to have good grounds for such an action. For some reason that I still cannot fathom, it seems all right to destroy it for very minor reasons if it has no soul and is not a person, in spite of its being "biologically human."

The humanists who don't believe in souls anyway have an easier problem to solve: They just say if the baby is not wanted by the maternal host, or if it is not a perfect specimen, then why worry about "a bit of tissue"? Well, it is a complicated, kicking, wriggling "bit of tissue," and as for not being "wanted," the waiting time for adoptions is *years,* and Sweden and Denmark and West Germany are importing babies from southern Europe to meet the demand. It seems to me that if the developing baby endangers the health of the mother or the food supplies of the nation then something may have to be done about it. But I would rather see women being a bit more responsible about what they do with their own bodies—and save my profession from getting into the nasty business of destroying life when we are trained to save life.

The second month of pregnancy can be a time of bewildering emotional instability. The placenta is manufacturing hormones at a great rate and this may have something to do with the irritability, moodiness, and tearfulness that make some women seriously contemplate having the pregnancy terminated even though they had longed for a baby.

From twelve to sixteen weeks the baby grows fast so that by sixteen weeks he is about three inches long and weighs about six ounces; tooth buds are forming; eyebrows and eyelashes appear; the flat little blob of a nose has developed a bridge; the larynx is firm cartilage; and the skin, though it is transparent and the blood vessels can be seen through it, is beginning to thicken. The fetus can bend and twist and turn somersaults: Like an astronaut in space, he is weightless.

At twenty weeks, the baby weighs about one pound and becomes legally recognized as viable (i.e., able to live). At this time many countries require the birth to be registered if it occurs early, though there is little chance of such a tiny baby surviving because the brain and lungs are too immature to manage away from the mother's blood that supplies the nutrition and oxygen. Before this time termination of the pregnancy by accident or design is abortion.

By twenty-four weeks the length is only twelve inches and the weight is between one and two pounds and the baby is still very unlikely to survive if born prematurely. In fact, a baby of twenty-three weeks is the earliest on record to survive. At this stage his body is covered with fine hair (lanugo) and the skin is less transparent, though the vessels can be seen through it; the

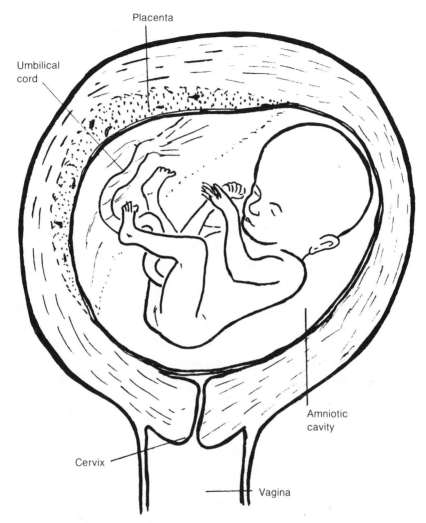

Placenta

Umbilical
cord

Amniotic
cavity

Cervix

Vagina

Actual size of fourteen-week fetus

fingernails and toenails are now well developed; and a soft fine
cream (vernix) appears all over the skin, secreted from glands in
the baby's skin. This is to protect the skin from getting
waterlogged as the baby swims in the amniotic fluid. He still has
plenty of room to move about and the mother can feel frequent
movements now, but he has periods of sleep and may be quiet for

hours. He is so clearly an identity that he now has his own fingerprints, though I doubt if any exist on police files at this age. Like the old advertisement for a well-known automobile, he floats on fluid—about two quarts of it. He is breathing fluid in and out of the lungs and has been known to get hiccups.

By twenty-eight weeks his eyes are open, he is about fourteen inches long, and about two pounds in weight—now definitely regarded as viable. He can hear; in fact some women say they can't go to concerts because the baby objects! Maybe he just objects to her sitting in one seat all night, but it can be proved that he can hear. If a bell is rung and he is poked to move, he can develop a conditioned reflex to move when he hears the bell without waiting for the poke.

The Child in the Womb

By thirty-two weeks he weighs over three pounds, measures sixteen inches long, and is beginning to get a little pad of fat under the skin. He is still a scraggy little object, but the lanugo is beginning to fall out and he has a fair chance of survival if he arrives then. He may suck his thumb if it gets near his mouth and he is getting ready to eat. The amniotic fluid is a little less and it is easier to feel the baby; besides, he is beginning to find it a bit more difficult to move about; his accommodation is getting cramped and he may stay in one position for quite long periods. He can't somersault any more, but he can kick and punch. Usually he is head down, and the doctor will probably tell you the position he is in when he examines you, and he may let you hear the heartbeat through his stethoscope. If the baby is tail down (breech presentation), the doctor may prod him to try to make him move around: Head first is the best way to face most of one's problems and labor is no exception. If he won't be moved fairly easily he will be left in the breech position in case it is a short cord that is holding him; and if the doctor thinks that it may be too risky for you to have your first baby this way, then he may decide on a Caesarean section, a very safe operation these days.

In the last two months the baby gets a good deposit of fat under the skin, his bones calcify more, he stores up some iron for blood manufacture after birth, and the skull bones hold the brain more firmly. His blood is changing over from fetal type hemoglobin to adult type, and it's all systems go! He is ready to be born and to manage independent life without trouble. Very critical for this is the development of the epithelium in the lungs: The baby's existence depends on whether he can breathe and use oxygen, and no amount of respirator assistance can make his lungs use oxygen if they lack a fine lining fluid called surfactant. A recently introduced test (called *amniocentesis*) makes it possible, by taking a little fluid from the amniotic cavity and examining the substances in it, to determine if there is enough surfactant to enable the baby to breathe.

Amniocentesis is rarely done, but its precautionary use is becoming more frequent. It is neither difficult nor dangerous. Women who have high blood pressure or diabetes or some other reason for being brought into labor early may have this test to find out if it is safe for the baby. Amniocentesis is also done to find out if the baby is affected by Rh problems; and by this test it is also possible to detect some rare abnormalities in babies as early as twelve weeks. A needle is inserted through the abdominal wall and into the uterus and fluid taken off. Cells in the fluid will belong to the baby and the chromosomes can be counted; and the fluid can be examined for abnormal chemical substances.

It is during the last two months that most if not all of the antibodies against infection are passed across from the mother to the baby; he will therefore be immune to most of the common diseases that his mother has had, or been vaccinated against, for about six months after birth.

Well, it's a wonderful story, isn't it? From less than the size of a decimal point to seven and a half pounds, entirely nourished by mother's blood. Judith Wright says it better than I can:

> *You who were darkness warmed by my flesh*
> *where out of darkness rose the seed.*
> *Then all a world I made in me;*
> *all the world you hear and see*
> *Hung upon my dreaming blood.*

I always have qualms about talking to pregnant women about the fact that sometimes things go wrong; not all babies are perfect and some mothers need to take a great deal more care of themselves during pregnancy than others for the sake of the baby and themselves. A woman does not grow up and become a mature woman until she can put the welfare of another before her own desires; and for many, pregnancy is the first real test—though marriage should have made her realize this. One hesitates to give women cause for fear, but I think fear is best combated with knowledge and, knowing just what is involved in bearing a child, the mother can avoid some of the pitfalls. If problems do arise at least she knows she has done her best for the baby and accepted her responsibility. Father needs to understand what is happening, too, so that he can give the emotional support and encouragement a woman needs when she has to refuse an occasional pleasure that she would so much have enjoyed, but that might possibly have harmed the baby.

The Placenta

Let's have a look at the environment of the developing baby. Not so long ago, we used to believe that the placenta was a barrier between baby and the dangers of the outside world, that somehow it selected the good things baby needed and filtered out the bad ones and sent them back to mother to be disposed of. This sublime faith in the protective power of nature was shattered when Sir Norman Gregg showed that the German measles virus can cross the placenta; and then another Australian, Dr. William McBride, observed that thalidomide was damaging babies. Now we know that the placental barrier cannot select the good from the harmful and the main factor in determining what crosses it is probably the size of the particle.

Next, doctors began asking questions about the placenta itself. Why assume it is always perfect? Perhaps the filter can be a faulty one, perhaps the placenta can be too small or even be diseased. Many research workers are now studying placental function. From this work are coming tests for determining the health of the baby in the uterus, and we have become aware that a baby can be undernourished. Here again we used to believe that nature always put the baby's health first and drew on the mother's tissue to feed her baby. To a large extent this is true: Nature does protect the

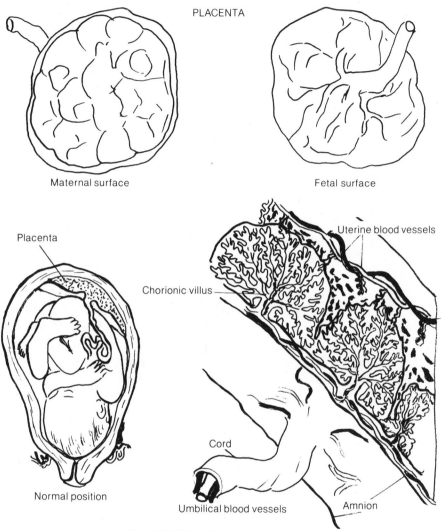

PLACENTA

Maternal surface

Fetal surface

Placenta

Normal position

Uterine blood vessels

Chorionic villus

Cord

Umbilical blood vessels

Amnion

PLACENTAL CIRCULATION

In the uterus the baby depends entirely on the mother to provide all his food and to remove waste products. The mother's blood is carried to the placenta by the uterine arteries, and the baby's heart pumps his blood along the umbilical vessels to the placenta to pick up oxygen and food. The bloods of mother and baby do not mix, being separated by a membrane. Note that the placenta is normally situated high in the uterus so that it will not cause any obstruction to labor.

baby from some unsatisfactory maternal care. We knew that in times of famine babies were smaller, but we believed that once they got the right food they grew fast and normally. Recent research has shown that a baby malnourished in the uterus does not catch up and may suffer permanent damage, including brain damage,—because the brain tissue is the most delicate and highly developed. It used to be said that some of the underdeveloped races were inferior; now thinking people are asking if this apparent inferiority in intelligence and physique is simply due to poor environmental conditions even before birth. The answer seems to be coming loud and clear that this is so.

The placenta is basically a huge folded membrane making up the filter, probably about a thousand square feet in area if we spread it all out, but folded down to the size of a round plate about eight inches across and less than two inches thick. On the maternal side where it is attached to the uterus it is spongy and bathed in maternal blood. On the baby's side it is covered with a thick membrane and the umbilical vessels can be seen entering and leaving it by the umbilical cord. There are two arteries along which the baby's heart pumps the blood to the placenta to get supplies, and one large vein coming back to the baby—the reverse of the situation as regards oxygen and blood vessels outside the uterus. Here the vein carries the oxygenated blood and the arteries bring back the carbon dioxide to be excreted by the mother, whereas in the mother the arteries are carrying the oxygenated blood and the veins are taking back the carbon dioxide to be breathed out into the air. The umbilical vessels are twisted all around the length of the cord and supported in a jellylike substance and surrounded by membranes to protect them. The cord is very variable in length (usually about two feet) and the twist in the vessels allows the cord to be pulled and stretched when the baby moves around, without any harm being done. Occasionally he ties the cord in knots, and sometimes it is too short; but these problems rarely cause trouble till labor starts and we have very reliable ways of detecting when the baby needs help, and we can rescue him. In the placenta the umbilical vessels branch so that there are about fifty sections of the placenta each with its own blood-exchange system. If one area of the placenta separates from the wall of the uterus, as it can in women who have high blood pressure, the rest may hold and keep the baby's needs supplied.

Drugs and Infections

Many mothers now worry about every dose of medicine they take and every cold they have during pregnancy; so I hope it will relieve your worries to know a little more about the noxious influences that *can* harm the placenta or the baby. Very important factors are the dose of the drug and the amount and severity of the infection. Nature takes good precautions where small doses are concerned, so we really only have to consider the organisms that are very dangerous even if only a few get through to the placenta, and the organisms that are very tiny so that a lot can get through. The same applies to the drugs. No one worries about one aspirin, but one thalidomide tablet at a critical time can do serious harm, and it appears that a lot of aspirin can too.

The common infections in the mother known to be able to damage the embryo and fetus are German measles, syphilis, smallpox, and the cowpox virus (vaccinia) used for immunization against smallpox. There are also a few very rare ones, some of which can cause infection in the placenta and disturb the baby's growth through interfering with the food supplies.

German measles in the first month of pregnancy can affect the baby in as many as 80 percent of cases, the figure falling to 10 percent when infection occurs in the third month and becoming less serious in its effects. Damage can occur to eyes, hearing, heart, brain, and kidneys. Between the third and fourth months acquiring the infection is unlikely to interfere with normal living; and if German measles occurs after the fourth month the majority of babies will be normal or likely to suffer only minor effects. Immunization against German measles should be done at least three months before contemplating pregnancy and there is now a test available to find if a woman is immune to German measles; this can be done at any time, including during pregnancy.

There is no evidence that immunization during pregnancy can affect the child, but it is not recommended because it does mean giving the mother an attenuated live virus. Vaccination against smallpox should not be done during pregnancy.

It is sound common sense for the pregnant woman to avoid contact with people with infections, particularly viral ones. Even if you have been immunized against measles, polio, and German measles, don't go and mind your friends' children who have the measles, and keep away from influenza, mumps, chicken pox, hepatitis, and nose and throat infections, particularly if there is a rash. These conditions are not known to cause abnormalities, but they are suspected of disturbing fetal nutrition. Herpes virus (the genital variety) is very common and can cause serious infection in the newborn baby when it is transmitted at birth, but it is very rarely thought to cross the placenta.

The whole situation with drugs is very confusing, and now all new drugs have to be thoroughly tested on pregnant animals of many different kinds before they are released to the public for use in illness. However, we do know that all drugs and medications given to the mother can be expected to cross to the baby in varying amounts, and some of these will be very big amounts for the baby since the dose was calculated for the mother. Our drug-oriented society pops a pill in its mouth at the slightest sign of discomfort and we simply do not think of the effect on the baby. Nevertheless, there are only a few drugs proved to cause abnormalities, and your doctor will guard you against these, whether they have been prescribed for some ailment (e.g., the iodides and other drugs used in thyroid conditions and asthma) or you feel prompted to take them on your own behalf.

In general it is wise to avoid taking medication, particularly in the first three months, except for iron and such medicines as the doctor considers necessary for health. On the other hand, medication is often in the best interests of the baby and very necessary during pregnancy. The woman in ill health is obviously not the best maternal host, and treating her condition with medication that does not harm the baby is good medical practice. The fetal abnormalities caused by faulty ovum or sperm are now thought to cause spontaneous miscarriage in most cases, and doctors are tending not to try to stop a spontaneous miscarriage. There is also some evidence that some inherited abnormalities are less likely to occur if the baby is given the best possible environment in the uterus. So don't imagine that all medicines do harm; the tablet that stops severe vomiting is important in ensuring that the baby gets his nourishment. Your doctor will reassure you about your indigestion mixture and occasional headache tablet. But do ask your doctor.

The substances that a pregnant woman really has to take precautions against are nicotine and alcohol. Both cross the placenta and both affect the nutrition of the baby. Alcohol in sufficient quantity actually damages the baby and a brain-damage syndrome has been described that can now be recognized as almost certainly due to large amounts of alcohol. Smoking aggravates the risk of raised blood pressure and affects control of the vessels in the placenta, thus reducing the baby's food supplies so that it is smaller than average. It is also much more irritable and pale and has a more rapid heart rate. Giving up smoking is not easy. You may get down to five a day, which is considered to do no harm, by timing the cigarettes and chewing something else in between; but father probably has to smoke away from home if he must, as two irritable, unhappy people do not provide the best environment for baby.

Abnormalities

A matter that has raised moral, theological, psychological and even public welfare issues lately has been the advance in science that has made it possible to diagnose the existence of an abnormal child in the uterus. It is possible now to diagnose mongolism and quite a number of the herditary metabolic diseases and some of the blood diseases such as hemophilia. This makes it possible to abort these babies even as early as twelve weeks, and obviously the techniques for diagnosing them will improve; and the law is unlikely to say that a woman who is carrying an abnormal child should not have the right to have an abortion. A professor of social medicine at a conference recently asked seriously whether this was not an unfortunate advance in medicine, because mankind preserves its ability to feel concern for others by caring for the disabled, and it will be a grim world that kills the aged and the ill and allows only perfect children to survive. On the other hand, an abnormal child can be a terrible burden for parents to bear. Maybe the answer lies in careful selection for abortion and better community services to assist those who have such problems.

6

What About
Breast-Feeding?

How are you going to feed your baby? This is a decision to be made before the baby arrives and a subject to discuss with your doctor. Being a pediatrician whose main interest has always been the first years of life and parent-child relationships, I suppose it is inevitable that breast-feeding should always have fascinated me. I became very personally involved when I had my first baby and accepted it as a matter of course that I should breast-feed him. I had been well indoctrinated during my medical course and believed that all I had been taught was correct: "regular four-hourly feeding," "no night feeds," "empty one breast before going to the other," and "get the cream," "ten minutes each side," "if there is not enough milk then complement with diluted cow's milk," "put him to sleep in his own room," "don't pick him up when he cries." Here I was, passionately loving my baby, wanting him near me at night, refusing to let him cry until his feeding was due or to give him boiled water in the night when my breasts were leaking milk. For me, rebelling against my teachers and becoming aware of their ignorance was a devastating experience. Modern students may take it more philosophically than I did but nothing satisfied me but to obtain a grant to do research on breast-feeding. After several years, I proved the correctness of my instinctive feelings. I studied the normal functioning of the let-down reflex and established the absurdity of some of the rules set down in textbooks. This led me to make contact with Dr. Mavis Gunther, Professor Niles Newton, and Dr. Harold Waller. They too were proving not only the nutritional value of mother's milk and the need to adopt scientifically based techniques for breast-feeding, but the importance of the psychological experience for both mother and child.

Old ways die hard, and there are still doctors who do not accept the fact that many babies are unable to tolerate cow's milk. They believe that as long as a baby gains weight, all is well—despite his protesting screams and his mother's despair over sleepless nights. But I am not happy about the routine use of diluted cow's milk. While I was doing research on infantile eczema, I discovered that in many of the babies given cow's milk, the eczema got worse. They also developed colic, and, often, vomiting and abnormal bowel movements. So I turned to processed milks, dried and evaporated milk, specially prepared formulas, predigested milks, acidified milks, and milk substitutes, such as soybean and goat's milk. I found them to be more satisfactory than cow's milk. I also found the modern bottles that allowed air in as the baby sucked and that had nipples to fit a particular baby's mouth to be much better than those that created a vacuum. Every year more substances are discovered that have to be added to the milk to make it more like breast milk; and the arguments about polyunsaturated fats, salt, and different sugars are, to say the least, confusing. But a mother need not worry if for some reason she has to feed her child with a substitute formula and with a container invented by man. Simply, having found breast-feeding a thoroughly enjoyable experience, and being convinced of its scientific value as nourishment for the baby as well as a part of the developing mother-child relationship, I have always wanted to help mothers breast-feed if possible.

I am always very pleased when I can advise a woman about breast-feeding during pregnancy rather than when she is already in trouble and has perhaps already weaned the baby. Both physical and emotional preparation can prevent many problems. However, it is an emotional subject. Women who have failed to breast-feed and nurses and women doctors who have not breast-fed a baby often tend to think the enthusiasts for breast-feeding an emotional, sentimental lot who overstress the subject; they maintain that artificial foods are just as good. Male doctors whose wives have not breast-fed their sons and daughters are often very much in favor of artificial feeding in a one-upmanship way. Start talking about breast-feeding anywhere and you soon become aware that you have stirred up the very depths of male and female mysteries. This is part of female sexuality (your husband will have feelings about it too) and you will find your attitude toward breast-feeding a test of your femaleness and mixed up with being a complete woman—whether you like the idea or not and whether you breast-feed or not. Women who do not like having their breasts fondled in lovemaking may not want to breast-feed. The busty beauties so beloved by magazines like *Playboy* and by those males that are afraid of deep commitment more often than not fail to produce the milk; whereas I have seen women who have a very modest bust endowment feed twins with great satisfaction. My son has a motorcycle for which I do not share his affection. He assures me that the sheer joy of riding a motorcycle makes all the hazards worthwhile and that I should not criticize bike riding or regard bike riders as crazy until I have tried it. He tells me that it takes practice, common sense, a sound knowledge of the rules, a good piece of equipment, and determination to succeed; that the dangers come from the crazy motorists who don't take care and the irritating critics who don't know what it's all about; and that the casualties mainly occur among the learners and there should be better teaching facilities. Well, that sounds like breast-feeding to me! I can only tell you why the milk is good for the baby and breast-feeding a joyful experience for me, and then you must decide for yourself, and I should like to help you.

The Scientific Whys and Wherefores

Nature has produced a different milk for every mammal, a milk to meet the needs of the little growing creature for the stage when his only food is milk. The little human mammal had largely become a parasite on the cow until science got going on the ingredients of baby food, but, as Oliver Wendell Holmes says, "The human mammary glands produce a more nutritious fluid than the two hemispheres of the most learned professor's brain."

Still, the scientists have produced some very satisfactory formulas. I doubt if they are really much better than what nature made for the kid and the calf as modified for human use, and they certainly taste a lot worse. Anyway, babies thrive on them, and if you can't produce the milk yourself then you need not worry about a suitable food not being available. With breast-feeding we are talking about something much more than mere milk, but you may like to know what changes are needed in animal milks to make them suitable for babies.

PERCENTAGE COMPONENTS OF ANIMAL MILK

	Human	*Cow*	*Goat*	*Buffalo*	*Horse*
Protein	1.1	3.3	4	4	2
casein	0.5	2.7			
lactalbumin	0.4	0.4			
lactoglobulin	0.2	0.2			
Sugar (lactose)	7.5	4.75	5	4	7
Fat	3.5	3.5	8	7	1
(saturated)	+	+			
(unsaturated)	+ +				
Minerals	0.2	0.75			

As cow's and goat's milk has to be pasteurized, most of the vitamins are destroyed and need to be added. In the early days of artificial feeding the formula was made up mathematically by adjusting the total protein, fat, and sugar—until it was realized that the fats and proteins were actually different; so now dried milks and "scientific" formulas take out some of the saturated fat and add unsaturated, reduce the calcium, and add more iron, to make the change nature wants for the human baby. After all, calves get out and eat grass quite early, and they have to stand on their own legs to do it; so they need less iron and more calcium in their milk. Babies fed on the higher-protein, higher-calcium formulas often gain weight faster and grow teeth earlier than the breast-fed; and though some competitive Western mothers take this as a sign of progress in their baby, who really wants heavier, toothier babies?

Knowledge of germs and better understanding of hygiene have

made artificial feeding safer: Mothers are now taught to sterilize bottles and prepare formulas very carefully, and there has been a very great reduction in the risks from infection such as gastroenteritis. However, the artificially fed baby who does get gastroenteritis is still sicker than the breast-fed one, and he also gets more colds. This has recently been explained by the discovery that the lactoglobulin in breast milk contains immunoglobulins that, given fresh, are not altered by the heating and drying process in preparing formulas. The immunoglobulins, like the vitamins, have to a large extent been named alphabetically immunoglobulin A, E, G, M, and they are all present in breast milk. The most interesting one is immunoglobulin A, which is the one that protects the mucous membranes lining the breathing passages and the stomach and intestines from infection, particularly viral infection. It is a very large protein particle, and it has been suggested that "it plugs the gut holes" and prevents other large molecules of protein from being absorbed into the blood too early and causing the development of allergic reactions.

Certainly breast-fed babies seem to have fewer allergy problems than the artificially fed, and it can be shown that antibodies against some foods do form in the baby's serum. Breast-fed babies can develop allergies, too, particularly if there is a strong family history of asthma, hay fever, hives, and eczema. We know that all kinds of food the mother eats do pass into the milk, but we can control these and advise the mother to give up eating eggs or drinking milk if we know she was allergic to them as a child, and we can make up any deficiencies in her diet with extra calcium and protein. There are also other substances in breast milk that protect against infection; in fact, so effectively that, when we give the attenuated virus of polio for polio immunization, antibodies from the mother may kill the virus, so that the baby should be immunized again after breast-feeding is finished.

Among other substances that go into the mother's milk are the hormones she is making in her body, or taking as the contraceptive pill, and substances like DDT that result from our widespread use of insecticides. Women breast-feeding should not take contraceptive pills, because most of them reduce the breast milk. There is a hormone that occurs in breast milk that may very rarely cause jaundice in the baby, but it is not a reason for weaning and is only temporary. There is no evidence that DDT in the quantities the baby is getting does any harm, and certainly its presence does not justify losing all the other advantages of breast-feeding. Obviously, though, it warns us that we should all be taking action against pollution of our atmosphere. There are other interesting substances in breast milk (such as inositol) in much larger quantities than in other milks, and we have yet to learn what their function is.

It has become apparent, since so many women in the developing countries gave up breast-feeding early in order to go out to work, that unsatisfactory artificial foods they may use can impair the development of the baby's brain and that the high-sugar, low-protein foods used in some of the poor areas may be affecting intelligence. This does not affect us in civilized countries where all the baby milks on the market are good, well-balanced formulas; but it is important to be sure the baby will tolerate such foods before weaning. It is advisable for babies with allergy-prone fathers or mothers to be breast-fed for at least three months if possible; but even a few weeks is better than nothing. It is the colostrum, or first milk, that contains the high immunoglobulin A; so even if you are going back to work early or don't like the idea of breast-feeding, at least start and give the baby time to find a suitable food. The protein of breast milk forms a small, soft, easily digested curd, very different from the large, hard curd or cow's milk. It is this ingredient, together with an interesting newly discovered one, lactoferrin, that influences the type of organisms that grow in the bowel and affect the smell of the movements, with the result that breast-fed babies and their diapers are sweeter smelling.

The Case for Breast-Feeding

Well, so much for the milk. What about the container? Can we really compare a hard glass or plastic bottle with a long, hard rubber nipple with nature's beautiful, soft, warm adaptable container that has a built-in let-down mechanism and a pulsating, comforting heartbeat behind it? Actually the baby has different sucking techniques for bottle and breast, and some recent studies have suggested that both breathing and speech can be influenced by the adjustment the baby's mouth and breathing passages need to make. Babies are extraordinarily adaptable creatures, and so are inventors of equipment; so the babies all learn to talk and breathe and the manufacturers go on studying nature and produce some really amazing nipples and bottles. But why not have the real thing?

What about the most important component of breast-feeding, the mother and her breasts?

Well, first let's straighten out some misconceptions. The average woman has the equipment and the desire to feed her baby and the vast majority of women can. Probably there is a hereditary factor, and just as we know there are good milking strains and bad milking strains among cows, so some women will not have as much milk as others—but they all have some. There are some reasons for not breast-feeding (more about them later) and some women have some mechanical breast difficulties, mostly correctable. Breast-feeding does not spoil the shape of the breasts; in fact it improves them unless you come from an African tribe that has not heard of brassieres and lets the children feed until three or four years of age.

Indeed, I wish that women who will not even try to breast-feed would decide the childbearing is not for them. I fail to see why any woman who will not care for her own child should still want to have one. It never seems quite fair to the child.

I am afraid I agree with Dr. William Cadogan, the founder of pediatrics, who two hundred and fifty years ago wrote, "I cannot help suspecting that wherever such neglect does exist, whether in regard to suckling or superintending the management of their children, and does not arise from want of health or from some equally warrantable objection, it can be charged on the depravity of the age, which insensibly corrupts the taste and perverts the judgment of many who wish to do well." Fashion has a very big effect on us and we are subtly led to believe that all new discoveries and products are good. It takes a woman of conviction to persist when she is having problems and her contemporaries are encouraging her to wean the baby. Have you ever noticed that most people seem to have a great urge to make others do as they do? If we breast-feeders are getting into the minority perhaps it is time we got up and declared ourselves and "demonstrated" in the modern manner.

A few years ago I supervised a little research study of breast-feeding, and some of the observations we made were on attitudes to breast-feeding. Of 144 women having their first baby, only 6 did not want to breast-feed at all, 2 because they disliked the idea, 3 for a medical reason, and 1 because she was traveling and had apparently been deluded into thinking the bottle would be easier while traveling. Of the others 93 were keen and the rest willing to start and see how they got on. Another study has shown that in Western society the two people who most influence a woman to breast-feed or not are her obstetrician and her mother; so if the first is an uninterested male and the second has failed herself you may not be getting the best influences.

Breast-feeding is part of the reproductive cycle. Menstruation, courting, intercourse, ovulation, conception, pregnancy, labor, and breast-feeding—all are associated with considerable changes in a woman's body and with strong emotional reactions. These emotional reactions are probably, partly at least, related to the hormone production and the variations during the cycle. During breast-feeding ovulation is reduced, actually suppressed at first. It is interesting to note from a research study that some women practicing the mucus-secretion ovulation method of birth control can tell when ovulation has started again and can suppress it by increasing the frequency of breast-feeding. The really interesting hormones are oxytocin from the hypothalamus and posterior pituitary, which is essential for the let-down of milk, and prolactin, which is present in the blood in quite large amounts for the first six weeks of lactation and is essential for milk secretion. Oxytocin is also the hormone secreted during labor to produce the contractions in labor and in orgasm, and it may be associated with the sense of relaxation and satisfaction following both labor and orgasm. Prolactin can produce mothering behavior in animals, so why not in women? We have a lot to learn about our hormones and our psyche yet.

Just as many women fail to achieve full emotional satisfaction in their sexual relationships, many fail to enjoy breast-feeding. A psychiatrist in the United States studying reasons for failure to breast-feed made the observation that 50 percent of the women who weaned their babies early by choice, or who did not start to breast-feed, also gave a story of poor sexual adjustment in marriage. It surprises me to hear women sneer at breast-feeding and openly state they found no pleasure in it and that artificial feeding was much more satisfactory because "only a fool ties herself down."

I do not hear these women boasting about their failure as lovers, though the unhappy marriage state of many of them suggests the sadly true situation. I am sure that many emotionally immature girls who are insecure in their role of woman will benefit enormously from successful breast-feeding, just as many women say that it is only after the birth of their first child that they fully enjoy sexual intercourse. Successful breast-feeding can influence this adjustment too; and I say "successful" because a further failure in the woman's role is very damaging to the morale. My study also showed that the women who failed the first time did not try the next time unless they were very determined.

Breast-Feeding Is an Art to Be Learned

Breast-feeding is an art that is learned, and when a woman fails to establish breast-feeding it is most often because she has not been shown the technique or been helped sufficiently. Not many girls these days have seen babies breast-fed at home and learned how. We slip off in private, and if we do try to feed a baby in public our sex-conscious Western society degrades the action as offensive. There have been newspaper reports of the law descending on a woman feeding her baby, and embarrassed men, who don't bat an eyelid at a topless barmaid, blush at the sight. So technique has to be taught in maternity hospitals by staff who know their job and take time to explain, encourage, and answer questions, and who give talks before the baby arrives and show women how to prepare.

Even doctors and nurses who encourage breast-feeding often make it a fussy, exacting task rather than a joyous coming together of two people learning to love each other. Like all other love affairs, it has its difficult moments. Sir James Spence knew what he was talking about when he said, "Every woman has to fall in love with her baby." Many do experience love at first sight when they see that greasy, crumpled object as it enters this world loudly protesting, but much more often love grows gradually. Baby is having his very first experience of love, and Bowlby and

other psychiatrists have shown that this development of attachment to another human being in the first year of life is critical
to emotional development. How much simpler and more pleasant
if the attachment is also physical and to the mother. Love, be it
erotic, maternal, or an affectionate response to need, requires
practice, discipline, unselfish giving, and some response from the
beloved. Many women need to get a smile from a month-old baby
before they really feel like a mother; hungry sucking is not
enough. If a woman has never really experienced love before,
what better time to learn all about it than with a baby at the
breast and maternal feelings flooding her being? But past experience is still a very real factor in success or failure. The
fathering a girl receive influences not only her attitude to men but
this area of womanly adjustment too.

Speaking of father, here is another word from Dr. Cadogan,
writing of a different age with different customs, but concerned
with the age-old story of man, woman, and child: "I would
earnestly recommend to every Father to have his Child nursed
under his own Eye, to make use of his own Reason and Sense in
superintending and directing the Management of it; nor suffer it to
be made one of the Mysteries of the Bona Dea from which men are
to be excluded." How modern, when we are urging fathers to
come to preparation-for-parenthood classes and to be present
during at least part of labor!

Research workers have shown that the main factors in successful breast-feeding are preparation beforehand, mainly in
desiring to breast-feed and becoming accustomed to handling the
breasts, and good supervision and nursing assistance in the
maternity hospital and in the first six weeks after the birth of the
baby. The baby's life is no longer endangered by insufficient milk,
but his emotional development may be upset by a howling, windy
few weeks and a messy, confused mother-child relationship. We
want to get off to a good, working mother-child relationship, and
it takes six weeks to establish breast-feeding securely.

Preparation

The preparation necessary is very simple. First, decide that you
want to try to breast-feed. If possible see a friend feed her baby

and get an idea of how to hold the baby and see how he sucks, a beautiful rhythmic movement, which allows him to suck and swallow then breathe through his nose when he needs air. See how she makes him let go without pulling him off.

If you have soft, fine white skin, or if you are a redhead, you may have problems with tender nipples, and it can help to expose the nipples to a little sunlight and toughen them up a bit. We all have skins that have been overprotected in this area.

The most important preparation is to wash the nipples once a day without soap. Remove the crust of milk that may form on the nipple after the fifth month and gently pull the nipples out to loosen them up, using some Vaseline or oil to replace fats removed in washing. Milk, or rather colostrum, will ooze from the lacteal sinuses under the areola as you press on the area, and this opens up the fifteen or twenty ducts that deliver milk to the surface. Buy a front-opening brassiere with wide adjustable shoulder straps at about five and a half months when the breast tissue has almost fully developed, and keep it well adjusted so that the breasts are held up and not allowed to drag down out of shape. It is a good idea to acquire the knack of expressing milk from the breast before the baby is born. It is much easier to learn this before the breasts fill with milk a few days after the baby arrives; and you may find it useful if you overfill later, or if the baby is not sucking very well. Don't brush the nipples or put alcohol on them; this toughens and hardens the skin and the skin may crack.

Ask your obstetrician if you can have the baby to the breast soon after delivery, for the baby sucks well then, and it is best for him and you if he has his first lesson within a couple of hours of arrival. He may be too tired and it may not be allowed; but no harm in asking, and it may be a great help. This gives you a good chance to have a look at him too. Make sure that the doctor and the nursing staff know that you want to breast-feed and make sure that the obstetrician has checked your nipples again a few weeks before you are due. He will have examined them at your first visit, but the nipples grow with hormonal stimulation during pregnancy, and small, even inverted, nipples may come out quite satisfactorily. If they do not, then there are special plastic or glass nipple shields that can be worn inside the brassiere that will help the nipple to come forward, and also to improve its shape if it is turned inward. Inverted nipples are hard to correct later and a little treatment beforehand is worth hours of it later.

Breast-feeding is not something that comes by instinct or even naturally these days. It needs some conscious effort in preparation and learning the technique.

Breast-Feeding Is
Not Always Best Feeding

There are several instances in which you should not attempt breast-feeding: if you have had tuberculosis within five years, if you have a malignant disease, or any severe chronic illness, or if you have a condition for which you are taking medication (as much of it goes into the milk). Diabetics are often unsuccessful in breast-feeding, but there is no reason not to try. Mothers who have had thyroid problems often have difficulty breast-feeding, and it should not be attempted when the mother is taking certain thyroid drugs. Epileptics, too, may not succeed, and in any case the drugs will be transferred to the baby. Finally, if there is very little breast enlargement, severely inverted or cracking nipples that will not respond to treatment, or eczema around the nipples, it is not worth continuing with breast-feeding.

If you do decide not to breast-feed your child, the hospital staff will give the baby either plain water or glucose and water the first day, and perhaps some pooled breast milk from the milk bank on the second day. If they hesitate to start on a diluted artificial milk they will then work gradually onto a scientifically prepared formula. These formulas have vitamins and often some iron added. The amount is calculated according to the baby's weight and then adjusted to his appetite. While you are in the hospital you will give him his bottle and learn the technique of making up the formula and handling the bottle as well as how to sterilize it to reduce the risk of infection. Your baby need not feel deprived of any love and affection as long as you hold him in your arms while you feed him, and give him as much attention and physical closeness as you can without actually having him at the breast. The aim is to give the baby the feeding that suits both mother and child best. Although the baby's needs must be the main consideration, they can be met without impairing the mother's ability to display affection for her child.

7

Woman in Labor

At our classes for expectant parents there is always a father who gets up and asks, "How do I know when to take my wife to the hospital?" Father thinks that is something he can be responsible for, but it is open to question and dependent on his state of mind. An ambulance or taxi could be safer. A taxi driver who did not know Sydney very well actually took me to the wrong hospital with my second pregnancy, so perhaps it would be wise to phone an ambulance or have a reliable neighbor on call.

The Beginning of Labor

As the time approaches you may get some hints. The estimated date of nine calendar months and seven days from the first day of the last period is as close as the doctor can get; but in the last week or so he may say, "The head is in the pelvis" or "The head is engaged," meaning that the baby is head downward as expected and is moving into position for delivery. You may also have noticed that you have "dropped" and are not carrying all before you in quite the same style. However, this may happen a couple of weeks before labor starts if it is not your first pregnancy, or just as labor commences. In the last weeks you will also notice that painless contractions occur. You may have noticed earlier that when the doctor was examining the position of the baby the abdomen became hard and he had to wait until it relaxed; that was the uterus contracting, and as labor approaches you will often find that even walking about may bring on a contraction and a feeling of pressure low down. These contractions can gradually become more frequent and regular. Even if they are quite painless, regular contractions at five-minute intervals indicate that it is time to take the already packed suitcase and depart for the hospital.

Not all labor starts the same way. You may wake up in the middle of the night in a soaking wet bed and realize that the "waters have broken" (a brisk hemorrhage or rupture of the membranes has occurred). If this happens when you are out shopping it is even more dramatic, and I think that in the last weeks of pregnancy you should not be far away from home and help, alone. Probably the commonest way to start is to have a "show"—a discharge of a little mucus and blood, like the beginning of a normal period. The contractions may be painful and cramping from the beginning, but they are relieved by relaxation. If it is the first baby then you can wait until they are regular at ten-minute intervals; but if it is your second then, depending on how far you have to travel, go when they are regular. Waters breaking is an indication to leave for the hospital as soon as possible.

Arriving at the Hospital

When you arrive at the hospital you will be taken to the maternity floor, and as soon as the nurse has checked that you are in labor and all is going well, that your blood pressure is all right and baby's position determined, you get down to the serious business of being prepared. The nurse wants a specimen of urine to test, then you have a shower. It is important that the skin should be clean, and though shaving is not regarded as necessary, a few hairs may be removed. The bladder and bowel should be empty so that baby may pass through the pelvis with as much room as possible, and an enema is usual to wash out the bowel. Your pretty nightie is whisked away and a much less glamorous hospital garment is produced that you will not be at all concerned about messing up. If you are fortunate enough to be in a hospital with a first-stage room you may be able to wait with your husband in a comfortable lounge; you may walk about if your membranes have not ruptured or you have had no more bleeding than a normal show. There will be a couch or bed to lie down on if you wish, and a TV set; in fact, I have heard nurses say that they sometimes had trouble getting the mother to leave Dr. Welby or Dr. Kildare for the real one. From now on you can forget your modesty. For everyone around you this is all in a day's work; you are now the central figure with a job to be done and it can all appear a bit impersonal.

The nurse examines you, announces cryptically, "Two fingers dilated," and goes off to ring the doctor. She simply means the os, or opening of the uterus, is now far enough open to admit two fingers, and progress reports of "three fingers" and "fully dilated" will follow in due course. You may also hear that you are "ROA" or "LOA" or "posterior." These terms apply to the position of the baby, the most usual position being head down with the back toward the front so that it is easily felt on the right or left; if the back is toward your back then it is "posterior." Don't get worried if you hear your nurse remark to her friend with the next mother, "Mine is a primip, ROP, two fingers dilated, what's yours?" She is simply saying this is your first baby, in the second most common position, and that you are well on in the first stage.

The birth of a baby is a crisis experience, the culmination of nine months' preparation, a time of testing, the entrance to a new way of life; and I always think of these lines from Judith Wright's "Woman's Song":

> *Today I lose and find you*
> *whom yet my blood would keep—*
> *would weave and sing around you*
> *the spells and songs of sleep.*

So let us have a brief look at what labor involves. Your big questions are undoubtedly; How painful will it be? and How well will I manage?

The Stages of Labor

Labor is divided into three stages.

FIRST STAGE

In the first stage the contractions of the muscle of the uterus gradually dilate the os (i.e., the entrance to the uterus from the vagina) until it is quite flattened out and the baby's head can move into the vagina. The pain of the first stage can be greatly relieved by learning relaxation and attending a preparation course that relieves anxiety and teaches you what to expect. A study of the preparation-for-childbirth program in the hospital where I work showed that women who knew what to do in labor and approached it with the knowledge that they would be helped (even though they only learned the techniques of relaxation while already in labor) had a shorter labor than average and required less anesthetic and pain-reliever. This may not apply to the labor induced with synthetic oxytocin injections, which may intensify contractions and increase discomfort so that pain-relieving medication is essential though the labor may be shorter.

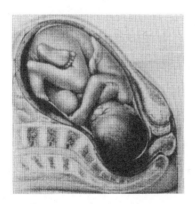 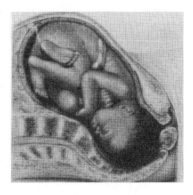

Normal labor: the first stage, up to the opening of the cervix

SECOND STAGE

The second stage is much shorter, two hours or less, even in the first labor, whereas first stage is often twelve hours. The second stage is associated with greater discomfort as the head is passing through the cavity of the pelvis and keeps up the stretching of the ligaments and the pressure on the tissues so that there is diffuse pain in between contractions. Pain-relieving medication is likely to be needed and is usually given before the mother enters this stage so as to provide relief throughout labor. In the second stage the whole process becomes automatic and inevitable: as one writer describes it, "like being caught in the rushing rapids of a river, buffeted about and finally so involved in the struggle for survival that nothing else enters awareness." Muscle relaxation between contractions conserves energy. Nature has already relaxed the ligaments; you know you can rely on your ob-

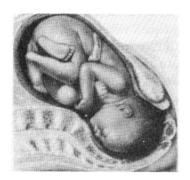
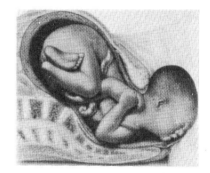
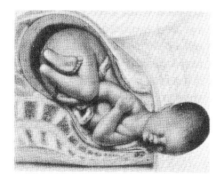
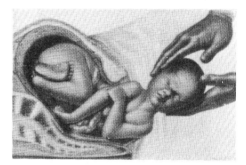

The second stage: the descent through the pelvis and the birth of the baby

stetrician, and all you have to do now is follow instructions. You automatically push down with each contraction and you will be told if the doctor wants you to let up on this push toward the end. Labor reaches a crescendo in discomfort and involvement as the baby is born. Few women go through the second stage without considerable discomfort, particularly at the beginning and the end, and relief is available according to your need; but doctors prefer to refrain from giving much medication because the baby also receives it through your bloodstream.

THIRD STAGE

The third stage is the expulsion of the placenta, when the uterus contracts again a few times, up to half an hour after the baby is out. The placenta separates from the uterus wall with some bleeding and is pushed out. Some women feel the contractions as painful; to others they are much less painful than the earlier ones, and the actual delivery of the placenta is not painful because the passages are stretched already.

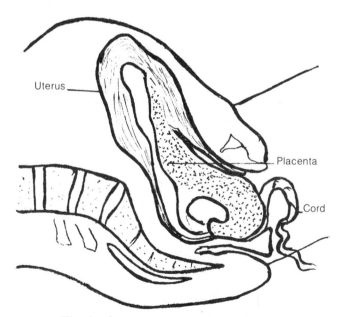

The third stage: the expulsion of the placenta

What About Pain?

Appreciation of pain is a very personal thing. Women tolerate pain better than men: No doubt nature made allowance for childbirth. Some women are much more sensitive to pain, and in some cultures it is permissible to express one's discomfort in sound and fury, so labor often sounds worse than it is.

Nature has two mechanisms for coping with the pain of labor: One is to blank it out if it is too great or to enable you to be distracted from it, and the other is to wipe it from your memory very soon. So don't be worried about whether you can bear it: Your relaxation technique will stand you in good stead. Don't expect that you will have a painless labor or think that you have failed in your preparations and your performance if you need help and pain-relievers. Primitive women have pain in childbirth, as Margaret Mead has shown, and my Siamese cat comes and tells me very reproachfully when labor starts for her. Siamese cats talk, and mine tells me that she does not have painless labors. I can assure you from my own four experiences that labor is a vastly satisfying, exciting, and triumphant experience. Discuss how you feel about pain and its relief with your doctor before you come into labor and you will have confidence that you will only get a pain-reliever if you want one and it will not harm the baby.

Childbirth is a time when what one really values in life seems to crystallize: to be loved, to love, and to feel you are a worthwhile person achieving something. The researchers say that this also affects the amount of pain perceived and the way a woman copes with it. If she feels loved and her husband is interested and wanting to help her, and if she looks forward to this baby as the fulfillment of their love, and sees herself as a woman with a purpose and a job to perform to the best of her ability, she has less pain, provided there is no complication. All women approach labor with some anxiety and fear. That is normal in the emotionally healthy woman facing the reality of birth. In these days of scientific obstetrics you are in no danger; and your baby's welfare is to be a major consideration in your treatment.

May Father Come In?

Your husband can be a great help supervising the relaxation during contractions, but most hospitals will quite reasonably have insisted that he meet several requirements first, such as having attended some classes for expectant parents, promising to leave if asked, getting the doctor's permission, etc. In a busy hospital, particularly at night, you will appreciate having him there for the first stage at least. As the cervix becomes fully dilated you find it much harder to relax. Nature now automatically calls into action all the muscles needed and you feel you are part of the inevitable future of the second stage. You now have no choice, your task involves hard work, and you realize why it is called "labor." Some women still fight against fate and abuse their husbands and make a great noise; but knuckling down to the job soon gets results and you need to concentrate to relax between contractions. This enables you to conserve your energy and take pressure off the baby. At the beginning of each contraction you now take a deep breath and if the doctor says it is all right to push then push down with the contraction, taking another quick breath if necessary while still holding the push. It is a help to have your husband to guide you with this. At first you may want to push before the doctor allows it, but try not to until you are told; it saves your energy and gradually the bearing down is inevitable.

The Delivery Position

As the baby's head descends and presses on the bowel you may feel that it is opening, but don't worry, that is normal and the nurse may hold a warm, moist pad across the vaginal opening and ask you to push into her hand. By this stage the nurse will have got you into the delivery position and called your doctor, who will probably have been in to see you earlier anyway. The delivery position is a matter of great controversy. Some doctors like to have the mother in what is called the left lateral position; this is on your side with your legs held up by a nurse or a metal frame. This is easier for the doctor, though uncomfortable for the mother, and many doctors insist on this position for the first baby because it gives them much better control of the whole situation. For the mother it is much more comfortable to be on her back, and many are advocating a return to the position used by more primitive people, in Russia, and the East, the mother leaning back in a half-sitting position. You will be draped with sterile towels and have a dab of antiseptic cream around the perineum to reduce the risk of infection. Sometimes during the second stage you find that as you relax after a contraction you get the shakes; this is quite normal and you cannot control it. You may also have a strange sensation of not being there at all and waft into semiconsciousness. It may help to make faces and grunt and even call out, but don't let that worry you; everyone does it. It is sheer waste of effort to clutch the nurse and make a lot of noise. Hang onto the bed instead.

The Delivery

Before long you will hear the welcome statement that "the head is peeping" or "the perineum is bulging" or simply "the baby is nearly here." As the head is about to be born the doctor may tell you to stop bearing down so that it comes more gradually and is less likely to tear the skin as it stretches. By this time you will usually have had a few whiffs at the anesthetic machine as you feel contractions coming and may be wafting in and out of consciousness. In fact, those few breaths may be quite heavenly and not interfere with your being conscious at the birth as so many women now wish to be. You will feel that everything is about to give way, and you waver somewhere between "this can't happen to me" and "what the heck"—and then a voice says, "You have a beautiful daughter." There is no doubt about the ecstasy and relief and tremendous sense of achievement as your child is born. This is one of the great moments of life: You have fulfilled your destiny, you are at one with nature, and nothing else matters.

The Baby Is Born

It is usual to have an injection just as the baby is born. This is to make the uterus contract and prevent bleeding, and it may force out the placenta. In any case, the placenta soon separates, and just as you think that all is over and the first excitement of seeing your baby is still with you, you get another contraction. You may feel quite indignant, but it is soon over. You may have a few stitches then or later, with a whiff of anesthetic if necessary. Occasionally the placenta does not detach itself, and the doctor may have to remove it while you have a little more anesthetic.

If you have not already had a good look at the baby and let him have his first suck at the breast, this is the time to do it. The sooner you see father, the happier you will be, too—and then a wash, back in your own nightgown, and a well-earned, relaxed sleep.

Local Anesthetics

If you have been given an epidural block, a spinal anesthetic, or a pudendal block, the actual birth will not be painful, for these are all types of local anesthetics given to cut off the sensation of pain from the nerves in the area, and your experience of labor will be

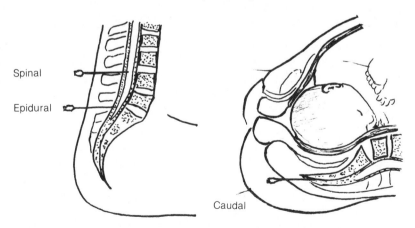

Position of needle in different types of anesthesia

different. An epidural anesthetic is given by injecting local anethetic into the lower back and affects the nerves just before they enter the spinal cord. It can be given in the first stage of labor, or a forceps delivery, or even for a Caesarean section. It not only temporarily removes the pain sensations, it makes the legs numb and heavy and powerless, prevents the bladder and bowel from working, and removes the other sensations of labor. It also takes some time for its effects to pass off and for normal movement and sensation to return; occasionally headache and some difficulty in passing urine occur for a short time. The baby is usually delivered by forceps because the mother cannot push it out. Many women consider that the removal of pain is the prime consideration; others resent the helplessness and feel frustrated. Some doctors want to use epidural block as a routine; others find it a very valuable method of pain relief when there are problems; in any case it needs an expert anesthetist.

A pudendal block is given lower down in the perineum or vagina and blocks off pain from the vagina; a spinal anesthetic is given higher in the spinal cord than an epidural one and requires more skill.

Possible Complications

A normal delivery is not for everyone. Nature may have intended childbirth to be a triumphant experience in a conscious woman, but science has enabled doctors to step in and save a mother and baby when things are not going normally. Your pelvis may be small, your baby big; the placenta may not be in the normal place; an episiotomy (a cut made by the doctor) may save a bad tear in a bad place; instruments can save a baby's life by hastening his arrival and that will need a deeper anesthetic; a Caesarean section may rescue a baby in distress. Anesthetics and forceps are great modern aids to safe obstetrics and have enormously reduced the pain and discomfort of childbirth and saved many babies from being damaged by lack of oxygen and labor that was too long; so don't underestimate their value in the hands of a good obstetrician.

The Movements for Normal Childbirth

The movements for normal childbirth must not be ignored. Dr. Grantly Dick Read removed a great deal of the pain from childbirth by removing fear, teaching women to relax between contractions, making sure that they were never alone, making sure they understood labor and their part in it. He made women members of the labor room team, fully involved, with complete confidence that their doctor would put the welfare of mother and baby before all else. He developed a preparation program, time-consuming for the doctor, but rewarding for both mother and doctor.

PSYCHOPROPHYLAXIS

Velvovsky, in Russia, Lamaze and Vellay, in France, developed the psychoprophylactic method of preparation, at first popularly called painless childbirth. This depended on the development of conditioned reflexes that reduced the mother's awareness of the uterine sensation and reduced pain. She learned to use her contractions and how to relax, but she also learned routines that she followed to send other stimuli to her brain, such as light abdominal massage; and she learned breathing patterns that helped her during labor. The emphasis was on learning techniques and being able to rest and reduce fatigue during labor. Psychoprophylaxis has helped many thousands, probably millions, of women. Some of its overenthusiastic supporters do not recognize that it is not suitable for all women, and most have now abandoned the term *painless childbirth* and there have been considerable changes in breathing techniques. Since the appreciation of pain is very variable, some do achieve a completely painless childbirth; but it is no reflection on the mother if she does not.

Many preparation-for-childbirth programs have now taken from both Grantly Dick Read and the psychoprophylactic teachers what seems most appropriate for the average woman;

they teach relaxation, correction of posture, efficient utilization of contractions, and regulation of breathing, with very successful results.

Induction of Labor

All the methods of controlling labor by preparation may prove hard to apply in a labor that has been artifically induced. Oxytocin is one of the normal hormones that the body produces to make the uterus contract. Until recently, one way to bring on labor was to put a very small amount of a synthetic oxytocin into a bottle of saline solution and let it drip into the bloodstream until contractions started. The uterus is very sensitive to this substance and the response was variable. Some women had much more forcible and painful contractions, so that they had difficulty in relaxing between them; others experienced a normal labor. Statistics show that the labor was shorter and more forceful. This could to a certain extent, be controlled by the amount of synthetic oxytocin used and by having someone with the woman all the time. Some hospitals used a routine strength—one unit or five units or ten units to the liter in the drip—and obviously this did not suit everyone. Constant observation of mother and baby was necessary to enable the rate of the drip to be varied.

The synthetic oxytocin drip was a valuable aid to modern obstetrics; but why was it used so much? For the convenience of the doctor? There was talk of 9-to-5 obstetrics, with a minimum of weekend deliveries! The current trend, however, is to allow the majority of women to come into labor naturally, when nature intends it. But statistics show that if the birth is two weeks overdue or there are some maternal ill-health problems the baby may be endangered, and an induction is then indicated.

Labor can also be stimulated by surgical means. The membranes are punctured by inserting an instrument through the os and releasing some amniotic fluid, then loosening the membranes around the os by stripping them from the wall of the uterus for an inch or so. This is a more certain method, but it has more risks than the oxytocin drip. It does not interfere with the uterine contractions.

The old-fashioned methods of taking castor oil or going for a rough ride on a bus are out.

As a pediatrician whose main interest has always been the newborn baby, I have frequently expressed anxiety that some babies were being pushed out too forcibly and that we could not determine whether there would be any long-term effects of their being rather more shaken up by birth than perhaps was necessary. Some seem mildly concussed, others seem more prone to jaundice. Other doctors are expressing doubt about the safety of increasing the force on the cervix, and suggesting that the labor may be more traumatic as well as more painful. Added to these doubts is whether an increased level of oxytocin is really the normal mechanism for starting labor and whether prostaglandins might not produce a more normal labor. On general principles, any alteration in nature's pattern needs very careful supervision and better indications for its use than the convenience of the doctor or the mother.

The Cultural Warping of Childbirth

In 1973 the International Childbirth Education Association in the United States published a booklet written by Doris Haire in which she very perceptively reviewed the whole problem of the "Cultural Warping of Childbirth" and its possible harmful effects on mother and child. The agitation for home deliveries of babies is not just a fad or a way of reducing hospital and doctor's bills; it comes from a deep-felt unease at modern methods that could plunge women back into the bad old days when the lives of mothers were lost through hemorrhage and shock and obstructed labor. Dr. Miller, working in a large obstetric hospital in San Francisco and commenting on the greatly increased demand for home delivery, says that though some of these women are "hippies seeing in childbirth an intensely beautiful mind-freaking trip" and prepared to risk a "bad trip" and even lose the baby for the sake of the opportunity to have a "good trip," mostly they are "intelligent thoughtful young people . . . training for childbirth, dignified childbirth with husband participation. I sense a growing hunger among young couples for more of this. They seem to know that as important as a good childbirth experience is, it is not enough to stabilize their lives and their marriage. They are anxious to learn how to make a man-woman relationship more meaningful, more permanent, more profound, more loving, and less hostile so that they can bring their child into a home un-warped by ancient plagues."

I am afraid the plagues are not all ancient; there are modern ones, and Doris Haire is right when she talks about cultural warping of childbirth. But the answer is not home obstetrics; it is team obstetrics and more appreciation of the personal needs of men and women and their babies. The obstetrician also has been caught up in the modern plagues, and he is in a very difficult situation when the woman demands a painless good experience, even if it carries risks for her baby and may disturb her normal psychological adjustment at the birth of her child. Childbirth is one of the all-consuming experiences of a lifetime and demands full involvement. Perhaps you can be a voyeur, putting your own comfort first to avoid the discomforts of really living. But there should be full involvement in the labor room, unless the life of the baby has to be saved by expert interference that requires full anesthesia.

Dr. Miller is making a very significant observation when he says that so many young people want to experience life and lasting human relationships; and surely the way to achieve this aim is to study the fortunate men and women who have happy, lasting relationships and are rearing their families joyfully and responsibly with ecstatic ups and agonizing downs.

The Husband-Wife Experience

The birth of a baby can bring a man and woman very close together as they share the experience of creating a new life and pledging themselves anew to rearing the child to the best of their ability. The hospital staff must be made aware of this, and they must respect the privacy and the sensitivity of the man and woman. Some women feel that they need the presence of their husbands right through labor; others prefer them out of the way and only want capable staff who know their job on the spot, but with father ready to appear as soon as the hard work is over and mother is restored to her normal attractive self—with an extra glow of achievement. Some men are a great help, others are easily distressed by the obvious effort involved and their inability to do much to help. Some, of course, just can't stand the sight of blood without keeling over or lighting a cigarette, neither of which is appreciated in a labor room. Then there is the man who must see his son born! It's probably a daughter, anyway, and he is wanted at the top end of the bed to comfort his wife not at the bottom obstructing the activity of the staff. The woman who wants "to make him see what I have to go through" is rather a menace, too, and this is not regarded as an adequate reason for having husbands present. The birth of the baby is a very personal and individual experience—some even want it on tape!—but, please, not at home.

Nature Versus Science

The aim and object is a healthy baby and a mother who is capable of looking after it and who is happy in her experience. In what we call "at-risk pregnancies," when either the mother or baby is at risk, then we need all that modern science can give us. When all is normal and proceeding as nature intended, then it is not a difficult business. The snag is that risks can arise at any stage of the pregnancy and delivery, so expert help should be at hand. Hence the system that has evolved in most civilized countries of a midwife or general practitioner caring for the mother and delivering the baby either at home or in a hospital, but having available the services of obstetricians and hospitals with high-powered modern aids. As the first birth is more likely to encounter problems, it is now usual for a woman to have her first baby in a well-equipped hospital, and certainly any woman who has had previous problems or in whom problems arise during pregnancy should have close supervision and skilled medical help in a hospital. The second pregnancy is the safest, then the third and fourth, but statistically the fifth carries the same risk to mother and child as the first.

It is quite obvious that the solution to the nature-versus-science problem is that the hospital obstetrics must provide more natural surroundings and interfere less with normal labor. With my main interest being neonatal pediatrics, I have observed the obstetric scene for twenty-five years and have become increasingly concerned as I have seen obstetrics become a branch of surgery greatly influenced by American teaching. The delivery of a baby is not a surgical operation unless serious problems exist; nor, as some women seem to think, is it an episode that the doctor manages while the patient sleeps or has pain completely removed. Child psychiatrists and pediatricians interested in baby care are becoming aware of quite serious disturbances in mothering behavior that may have their origin in pregnancy and childbirth, particularly if the mother has had a poor example of mothering from her own mother.

The Importance of the Delivery Period

Two critical situations or relationships seem closely linked with the experience of childbirth.

First, the establishment of the mother-child relationship: The confidence and joyfulness with which the mother accepts her child and feels an ability to provide its needs is certainly influenced by the birth experience. Secondly, the child's first experiences after birth can be expected to influence his personality development.

It is therefore essential to regard the delivery period and its management as a very important time for both mother and baby, and to regard the staff, both doctors and nurses, as members of a team to guide these two through the critical transformation from parasitic to individual life for the baby, and from incubator to active motherhood for the woman. It is unfortunate that women have come to look on the birth of a baby as a kind of illness because of the conditioning they have been subjected to by doctors and hospital staff. As Doris Haire says, they have become too submissive in accepting the patterns set for them. Women hailed Grantly Dick Read with thanks for including the mother as a person in the team, and with their new sense of importance in the world they may well have to insist on change. But women are divided in their wishes: The woman wanting to escape from her womanly role is apt to demand an epidural block, a short labor, and someone to care for her child as soon as it is born; whereas the woman who wants to be fulfilled as woman the person, the mother, and the wife is demanding to be fully participating, conscious, and triumphantly successful with her husband by her side and her baby to her breast as soon as it arrives. But the majority still just do as they are told in traditional fashion and take what comes for better or for worse. Dr. De Lee, the writer of a standard textbook on obstetrics, says, "The way to meet women's demand is not to give them more anesthetics, but to use less and educate women's minds."

A French obstetrician, Frederick Le Boyer, recognizes birth as an intense experience for the baby who is forcibly pushed into a cold, brilliant, noisy world. Le Boyer dims the lights and softens the sound. The baby is gently placed on the mother's warm, bare abdomen—even before the cord is cut—and then put into a comforting warm bath. A baby is treated as a sensitive person dangerously emerging into a new world.

Rebellion

There is a strong rebellious move, particularly in the United States, against so much medical interference with what people expect to be a normal, natural event, not an illness. Women complain bitterly that they have prepared for a natural childbirth, then arrive in the busy impersonal atmosphere of the maternity hospital and are swept into a machine over which they have no control. They have drugs and anesthetics they did not want and wake to find they have missed all the excitement; they complain in some hospitals that the nurses chase their husbands out, leaving the mother alone with a bell that she dares not ring; they also complain that they may not get their hands on the baby for hours and that to get it onto the breast soon after delivery is a major feat in most hospitals.

Women are rebelling against the very common practice of making a cut (episiotomy) to avoid a tear in the perineum, against lift-out forceps, against induction of labor. They find themselves involved in hospital routines and wonder if their doctor is also so caught up in the machine that he is perhaps unaware of the medication that is given. They want minimal or no shaving, since it has been shown to be of no advantage; they want less medication, more company and supervision to relieve apprehension, some light refreshment during labor, since hunger and hard work don't go together very well and the baby's blood sugar may fall; no induction of labor unless medical indications exist, no delaying the birth until the doctor arrives, no anesthetics that make forceps necessary.

Obviously all this needs discussion with your doctor well

before you come into labor. Don't say you don't like to take up his time. He is being well paid for it; this is one of the big events of your life and all in a day's work for him. It is time women stop being submissive creatures and actively and intelligently cooperate in labor with full knowledge of what is happening; and it is time they cease to regard the obstetrician as some sort of god.

Some women are delighted to be able to choose the baby's birthday and avoid the doctor's vacation by having an induction. (Somewhat confusing for astrologers: Can we now choose a zodiac sign for the baby, or will the astrologer need the date as estimated by the doctor and then corrected according to the mother's ideas of the day of conception?) Some women virtually demand a painless labor and an epidural block. I heard one recently say it was marvelous: She discussed the Vietnam war with the doctor while he applied forceps to the baby she could not push out because of her epidural block and she did not feel anything at all. This is devastating to a woman who wants to be involved. Do this to a sheep and she will kick the lamb away and refuse to accept it. Have some of the women who demand to be relieved of all pain and who force the doctor's hand already rejected the child and set a limit on what they are prepared to do for him?

Modern Aids to Safe Delivery

If problems arose during pregnancy it used to be the doctor's experience that guided him, for there were very few tests that could tell him what was happening to the baby. The fetal heart could be heard, and if movements were active and the baby was growing normally then it had to be assumed that all was well. However, sometimes the baby stopped moving, or became overactive, or the fetal heart varied in rate; sometimes the mother developed high blood pressure or had some bleeding or passed protein in the urine; and the doctor had to decide whether he should bring her into labor early and risk the dangers of prematurity for the baby.

Some years ago X rays were used quite extensively to determine the size of the pelvis, the position of the baby and placenta, and how many babies there were; but doctors became wary of the effect of X rays on the fetus and kept their use to a minimum. It is important to know where the placenta is in the uterus, and various methods were devised that showed it up by using X rays or radioactive isotopes; but these too were not without some risk.

The majority of labors are normal and do not require high-powered science; but let me tell you of some of the tests that can now show us what is happening to the baby while he is still in the uterus.

ULTRASOUND

In recent years a very safe method of using sound waves is enabling doctors to determine what is happening inside the uterus. An ultrasonic device maps out the structures in the uterus by projecting sound waves across the uterus, and these are reflected from the surfaces they hit. The reflections are seen on a screen and can be photographed. The doctor can thus see whether the placenta is in the upper segment of the uterus, where he likes it to be, or whether it is on the lower part or even across the opening; he will also be able to tell if there are twins. If there has been bleeding during pregnancy or there are doubts about the size of the uterus being what is expected, then this test may be done. It also determines the size and growth rate of baby's head.

A new harmless method of finding the position of the placenta is by *thermography*, which measures temperature change.

URINARY ESTRIOL

Another useful test is the determination of urinary estriol. So long as the mother is passing normal quantities of this substance in the urine it is fairly sure that the fetus and placenta are safe and well, and the doctor can carry on treating a problem in the mother and delay starting labor; for estriol is mainly derived from a substance formed in the adrenal gland of the fetus. This substance goes through chemical changes in the liver of the fetus, then passes across the placenta to the mother again, where it is chemically changed in her liver and filtered into her urine through the kidneys, which also make some of the final substance, conjugated estriol. Most of it comes from the baby, and about 10 percent from the mother; the final estriol figure depends on baby, placenta, and mother. If the baby is ill or has some particular deformity or dies, or if the placenta is not functioning properly or becomes separated from the wall of the uterus by bleeding, then the estriol levels fall. Toxemia, high blood pressure, kidney failure (when small quantities of urine are passed), or liver damage in the mother will reduce excretion of estriol.

This test is likely to be done if the mother has toxemia, raised blood pressure, diabetes, a history of problems in previous pregnancies, or bleeding in the last three months, or if the baby seems small or is past the expected delivery date. Mainly it reassures the doctor that the baby is well by giving normal or high levels, but when the estriol level is low the doctor has to decide why it is low and whether this indicates the need for induction of labor or even a Caesarean section.

The urinary estriol is being estimated more frequently than it used to be and some doctors suggest that the time will come when estimations are done in all pregnancies at about thirty weeks and again at thirty-six weeks. Estriol also appears in the amniotic fluid and can be estimated if an amniocentesis is being done.

AMNIOCENTESIS

Amniocentesis is another valuable test introduced in recent years. A needle can be inserted after local anesthetic through the abdominal wall into the cavity of the uterus and a sample of amniotic fluid drawn off and examined. The main value at first was to determine whether there were bile pigments and Rh antibodies in the fluid, showing how severely an Rh-positive baby was affected and whether it needed a transfusion while still in the uterus. It was more helpful in these patients if it showed that the baby was quite well and Rh-negative too; then it could go right to term and not have to face the risks of prematurity. Now the test is also used early in pregnancy if mongolism or an inherited metabolic disease is suspected.

Another very useful test of the amniotic fluid has been the determination of the quantities and ratio to each other of sphingomyelin and lecithin. These, and the ratio of these, gives a reliable indication of the maturity of the baby's lungs, since they are the chemicals concerned in making a substance known as surfactant, without which a baby cannot develop normal breathing. Respiratory distress due to lack of surfactant is the main cause of death in premature babies. If it is not present then every effort is made to keep the baby in the uterus longer, and cortisonelike substances can be given to the mother to hasten maturity.

FETAL HEART MONITORS

Methods have been devised for recording the baby's heart rate and heart sounds while it is still in the uterus. Instruments known as phonocardiographs or sonocardiographs, using ultrasonic energy, enable us to hear and record the fetal heartbeat, count it, hear if it is irregular or too fast or too slow. A fetal electrocardiogram can also be observed, and this can be recorded either from the mother's abdominal wall or by attaching an electrode to the baby's scalp, which gives a more accurate picture. If either of these methods of fetal heart monitoring is being used it is also essential to record at the same time contractions of the uterus, because they affect the welfare of the baby. During contractions, the oxygen supply is reduced normally without any harm to the baby and probably does some good, since it gets the baby ready for the big change to breathing by itself. But if the baby is in trouble, then the contractions aggravate this and the birth may need to be hastened. So long as the fetal heart rate is normal all is well with the baby as far as labor is concerned.

BLOOD TESTS

Another way of determining whether the baby is having problems with lack of oxygen is to take a sample of blood from his scalp. This is done through an instrument called an amnioscope inserted through the cervical opening during labor. A small nick in the scalp enables a sample of blood to be collected and a chemical test of the acid-base balance in the blood is done. This test is done when it is suspected that the baby is in trouble. All these mechanical tests can only be done in well-equipped major hospitals and are done only if there are complications of some severity, or in research.

8

The Baby

I hope that obstetricians will not resent my invasion of their male-dominated world of obstetrics and my criticism of some of the modern, mainly British and American, methods that have been introduced into the management of labor. A laboring woman is completely dependent on those caring for her. Her dignity, her self-esteem, even her identity are threatened. Her talents, her beauty, and her self-possession seem of little use to her in labor, so she is hypersensitive to the remarks of those around her. If their comments seem to imply criticism of her or dislike or even contempt, the three great needs, to love, to be loved, and to feel like a worthwhile person, are seriously threatened.

Unmarried mothers have often told me with some bitterness how they felt or imagined they felt the contempt of some staff members. They felt they were treated without any consideration of their feelings; their babies were safely delivered, but the psychological experience was more traumatic than it need have been. Doctors and nurses do not always realize that the unmarried mother already has usually been through the experience of loving and finding she has been made use of and not really loved; of discovering that the man does not regard her highly enough to commit himself to the care of their child or even to see that she is cared for. She has taken the courageous decision not to destroy the unborn child and perhaps the even more courageous one to give it to an unknown family in adoption. Or she may have carefully considered her assets and what she has to offer a child in the future, and she may have decided to keep her baby. Whatever the decision, she is facing labor under much greater stress than the woman who has a husband who loves and respects her and whose child they both want.

In Australian hospitals I have seen a great change in the staff attitude to women in labor—more kindness, sympathy, and understanding from the nurses. At the same time I have noticed increasing resentment among nurses at the doctors' interference with normal processes: at the number of inductions, episiotomies, and elective Caesarean sections, at the amount of medication. As I lecture to nurses on the care of the newborn I often find it hard to support even some of my pediatric colleagues who seem to think they or a nurse can look after a baby so much better than its mother that she is not allowed even to touch it. Some even say that a baby must prove he can swallow by sucking a bottle of water before being allowed on the breast, that he should be wrapped in a metallic sheet to keep him warm rather than be held in his mother's arms.

Let us have a look at what babies want from life right from the beginning. This is my field of knowledge, and here again I think that the baby's interests should always come before those of doctor and nurse, and even before those of the mother as long as her life is not in danger. There are emergency situations in which the mother just has to accept that her baby needs expert scientific help fast, and her need to see and touch her baby has to take second place.

Labor and the Baby

Labor has been a strenuous experience for the baby as well as the mother. Uterine contractions are very powerful, and I doubt if anyone is ever pushed around in this world like that again. But the pressure of the contractions has its value. The intermittent pressure on the blood vessels temporarily reduces oxygen supplies and prepares the baby for breathing oxygen himself; the chest is compressed and amniotic fluid squeezed out of the lungs so that air can come in as soon as the baby breathes. One of the problems of Caesarean section is that the baby is born with lungs full of amniotic fluid that has to be emptied and sucked out very quickly.

During labor the baby's head is gradually molded to fit the shape of the mother's pelvis as it passes through. That may sound rather fearsome to you, but it is not: The baby's head is not one hard bone like ours; it is made up of several bones—frontal, parietal and occipital—which make the vault. These bones are formed by calcium being deposited in the thick membrane and they grow along the edges, unlike the bones that grow by forming cartilage and grow from epiphyseal ends. The skull then consists of sheets of bone set in membrane, and the whole brain is surrounded by this strong fibrous material. There is an inner compartment that separates the cerebrum from the cerebellum in the brain and supports them on a kind of shelf so that as the head is gradually compressed and shaped to pass through the pelvis the brain is protected by these membranes and bone. The edges of the bones can even overlap a little, and you may feel a ridge on your baby's head either across it or down the middle; this undoes usually within twenty-four hours once the pressure is off. You may also notice if you are very observant that the diamond-shaped space on the top of the head, known as the anterior fontanel, is smaller at birth than later on when the head fully expands again. This compression does the baby no harm; in fact, we often find that a baby who is shot out with great force very quickly in a "precipitate labor" in which the head does not have time to mold has more trouble than a baby who has been through a long labor and has had forceps applied to give the final pull to the head. In a forceps delivery the head may be very elongated, but it goes back to normal quite soon.

It is often possible for an observant midwife or doctor going around the nursery to tell from the molding of the head which way a baby presented at birth: the molding of a baby whose face comes out toward the back of the mother or toward the front (i.e., anterior or posterior); the baby that comes tail first (i.e., breech birth); the baby that comes face or brow first; and the Caesarean section baby with no molding. All have recognizable shapes, but they will nearly all end up with a head shaped like dad or mom or some remote ancestor.

The doctor will have checked the position of the baby many times and made sure that it is not lying across the mother's abdomen. During labor the staff will have been checking the position of the head and the way it is turning and bending forward. The baby is normally in a relaxed position with elbows and knees bent, all folded up into as small a parcel as possible so arms and legs don't get in the way; and careful watch is kept to make sure that the umbilical cord is not compressed. Occasionally the cord does get tangled and this is one of the main reasons for counting the baby's heart rate frequently: The heart rate is a good guide to a baby in trouble and an indication for action that can save it. You will be largely unaware of all this, but I think you should know what is happening so that you can cooperate, understanding how foolish it would be to refuse expert help.

Becoming a Separate Individual

In the uterus the baby has been getting ready for individual existence, and all organs are functioning, but some need to change their action when the umbilical vessels are cut. His heart has been pumping blood to the placenta where waste products are removed by crossing the osmotic barrier into the maternal circulation, and his blood picks up and takes back from the mother oxygen, glucose, amino acids, minerals, and some essential fatty acid. He has been breathing fluid quietly in and out of his lungs, and not much blood has been pumped to the lungs. As soon as the umbilical cord is cut the heart makes a rapid readjustment; it closes the opening between the right and left sides of the heart and closes off two big vessels, one that conveyed blood into the main venous system and another that allowed blood to bypass the lungs and go direct to the brain by connecting with the main arterial system. Now the right side of the heart has to pump blood to the lungs to pick up oxygen, and it returns to the left side of the heart and pumps from there around the body, delivering oxygen. The first breath of air the baby takes starts this anatomical readjustment, but the openings do not close completely at once.

The baby may take his first breath of air soon after the head is born, even though it may take another contraction to push out the body; and normally his first action is to protest loud and long about the treatment he has just received. That cry is the most exciting sound that ever comes from a labor room, or anywhere else for that matter. A new addition to the population announces his entry with a triumphant loud noise, welcomed by everyone; but from then on that cry is his means of communicating his needs and it demands attention. It is a disturbing, distressing sound that no one can tolerate for long without doing something about it. When I am taking classes with medical students on the care of the newborn and one of the babies starts to cry I am always interested to see who picks it up first. Often enough it is I, but usually one of the girl students quietly comes over and wraps it and props it on the left breast and goes on taking her notes. I prefer students not to take notes, but just to get the feel of babies and their problems; but note-taking is an incurable disease with students. Anyway the baby stops crying, and we go on. Observers of mothers and babies say that both left- and right-handed mothers put the baby over their heart, and probably the rhythmic beat helps to soothe him.

CUTTING THE CORD

When the baby is born he is still attached to the placenta by the umbilical vessels and while these pulsate he is still receiving oxygen from his mother. However, an injection of synthetic oxytocin or erogometrine is given the mother usually as the shoulders are born, and this makes the uterus contract. The main aim of this is to prevent hemorrhage as the placenta separates by keeping the uterus contracted down. It also has the effect of forcing the blood in the placenta across to the baby. In a completely normal uncomplicated birth, it was usual to wait until the cord vessels stopped pulsating, and this could take several minutes. An assistant kept a hand on the uterus through the abdominal wall and kept it contracted by rubbing, and in this way the blood got across to the baby, and the cord was then tied and cut. This blood can amount to one-third of the baby's whole blood volume and is important. This is also why the doctor keeps the baby down below the level of the mother after delivery, to let the blood flow into the baby, not back to the mother; so don't expect him to wave your baby in the air for you to see or to hand it to you before the cord is cut.

CHECKING THE BABY

The baby's first need is obviously oxygen, and normally the first powerful cry fills the lungs with air and we know he is over the first hurdle. It is important at this stage to assess the baby's general condition, and the best test of this was invented by a woman anesthetist, Virginia Apgar. At one minute after delivery, and again at five minutes, some observations are made on the baby. His heart rate is counted, and he scores 2 points if it is over 100, 1 if it is below 100, and 0 if it cannot be heard. His breathing is then observed: If it is good and he has cried, he scores 2 points; if it is slow and irregular, 1 point; if he is not breathing at all, 0. His muscle tone is next: If he is moving, active and firm, 2 points; if arms and legs pull up when stimulated, 1 point; if limp, 0. The reflexes present at birth are a good test of well-being, and if he responds with a cough or sneeze to having his nostril irritated, or throws his arms in the air at sudden change of movement, 2 points; if he makes only a mild protest, 1 point; and if no response, 0. If his color is nice and pink, the score is 2 points; if pink and blue, 1; if all blue or very pale, 0. So a perfect score in all these tests is 10 points.

Quite often the one-minute reading is not 10; but it is the five-minute reading that is important and indicates to the doctor whether this baby needs some special attention. If the score is under 7 he probably departs to the intensive-care nursery, where he can be watched carefully and have mucus removed or oxygen given if necessary, and also kept warm. This Apgar rating has proved a very useful method of sorting out the babies that have been a little upset by their birth, and a lower than 10 rating does not mean your baby is ill; it merely indicates that he needs special care.

Even before the cord is cut the doctor checks to make sure the airway is clear for the baby to breathe. He may have a mouth full of mucus or amniotic fluid that needs sucking out with a mechanical sucker. He is tipped upside down at about 45 degrees to drain out the mucus and amniotic fluid. If he has not already taken a breath, the handling and sudden cold air on his skin, the movement and the alteration in the oxygen and carbon dioxide in his blood, stimulate breathing.

Some doctors give a smack to stimulate the skin, but the old methods of hot and cold baths and strenuous stimulation are now recognized as likely to do more harm than good; and now we have ways of administering oxygen and artificial respiration if necessary.

SEDATION AND BABY'S BREATHING

The concern about giving the mother pain-relievers and anesthetics and sedatives arises from the fact that they can affect the brain centers that control breathing in the baby. For instance, when morphine was popular for a short time as a pain-reliever for the mother there was an increase in stillborn babies. Their breathing centers were so affected by the morphine, a powerful respiratory depressant, that they could not take their first breath. As a result local anesthetics have become more popular and doctors like to keep medication during labor to a minimum. It may be easier for you and the doctor if you have more sedation, but not for the baby, and it is surprising how most women relax and cooperate without a lot of medicine if they have someone with them and know what to do.

The baby has a million or so extra red cells per cubic millimeter and 80 percent fetal hemoglobin, different hemoglobin in its red cells from that of the adult. Hemoglobin is the pigment that carries the oxygen, and fetal hemoglobin can manage with a lower blood oxygen; so, though five minutes without oxygen could be fatal for an adult, the baby is safeguarded and can manage even for fifteen minutes without breathing, so the baby may not breathe at once. I never cease to marvel at the wonderful precautions nature takes. Over the next few weeks this hemoglobin changes over to the adult type to fit in better with breathing through the lungs.

CARE AFTER BIRTH

Once the airway is cleared and the cord cut, the baby is wrapped in a cotton blanket that has been warmed to body temperature; his skin is usually covered with creamy vernix that has prevented its getting waterlogged. It is not washed off but allowed to soak into the skin and grease it. Any blood and vernix around the eyes are wiped away, and any mucus in the mouth sucked out. The cut end of the cord is dabbed with alcohol to kill any germs, and then you are usually given a look at what you have produced. He may be plump, pink, and cherubic; he is more likely to be crumpled, greasy, and complaining—but incredibly beautiful and heart-stirring just the same.

At this stage the baby's sucking reflex is very active, and it is the ideal time to let him have his first lesson at the breast, not on a bottle. The technique is different, so why confuse him? Baby is usually sponged, just a quick cleanup so that he won't get cold, and then left for a few hours to sleep off the exhausting experience he has passed through. He has usually had his bowels open soon after birth, passing black sticky material called meconium. He has not had his bowels open before birth unless he has been short of oxygen and distressed, and the presence of meconium in the amniotic fluid is always a sign to watch him carefully in case he has inhaled some, so off to the special nursery for awhile! He has been passing urine in the uterus, so it may be a few hours before he passes more, but he now has to dispose of his own waste products; the mother had been doing this for him by taking them across the placenta.

The next physical need the baby will let us know about is that he is hungry, or rather thirsty, because it is fluid he will need first. This is usually given as glucose in water by bottle; and I am afraid that in Western-style obstetrics this is necessary for several reasons. In less sophisticated cultures the baby would be put to the breast at every whimper and get a little colostrum and that would satisfy him; but even if we do this the colostrum will probably not be enough, and the nipples may get sore from the unaccustomed stimulation of sensitive skin. The colostrum will not be enough because it is the practice in most hospitals to cut the cord very soon after delivery, and this means that some of the blood from the placenta does not get across to the baby; it may be only 30 or 40 milliliters, but this is enough to make the baby thirsty.

JAUNDICE

Another reason for extra fluid is that jaundice is very common in newborn babies and likely to be more so if the mother has received some anesthesia and medication, and labor has been induced by oxytocin; giving the baby extra glucose and water makes jaundice less likely. There are many causes of jaundice but the common ones are simply immaturity of the liver, as in babies born early, and temporarily disturbed liver function from medication or the stress of birth. What happens is that the hemoglobin from red cells breaking down in the bloodstream normally forms the pigment bilirubin, which has to be changed into a water-soluble bile pigment in the liver before it can be excreted in the bowel and urine. If there is a delay in the liver caused by lack of a special enzyme needed to do this, the baby may become quite yellow. The blood level of this pigment can be measured and if the unchanged bilirubin approaches a level that could harm the baby appropriate treatment is available. So if you suddenly find your baby with eye pads over his eyes and lying naked in a warm, brightly lit crib, don't get worried; this is quite a usual way of preventing the level from getting too high by the action of light on bilirubin. Exchange transfusion is now required much less frequently and usually only for Rh babies.

Adjustment to the New Life

During the next few days the baby has to adjust to individual existence outside his mother's body; he is a very helpless little creature with only a cry to tell us that he is not happy. His basic needs are oxygen, food, fluid, warmth, removal of waste, sleep, and a comfortable position. There may be some aftereffects of the birth and some minor difficulties in coping by himself. For instance, he may be irritable and restless and tending to vomit as if he had mild concussion—not surprising after such a bump on the head. Some babies actually have a bump to show you. A great many tend to posset (i.e., bring up some of their food) and all need to be kept warm. Most can manage to get sufficient oxygen from the air, but it is essential to lay them on their sides or front so that if a little milk does get vomited it does not interfere with breathing. One of the objections to "rooming in" day and night is that the baby does need close supervision during the night as well in the first few days, and it is a comfort to everyone to know that a nurse is doing a regular round of the babies and mother can sleep.

It takes a few days for most babies to accustom themselves to this new existence. There are a few scaly skins and there is a tendency to pick up infections such as "sticky eyes" and pustular spots and thrush, particularly if the mother has had some vaginal Monilia infection during pregnancy; but with a few antiseptic skin treatments at bath time and prompt treatment of any infection and alcohol applied to the cut end of the cord daily most babies go home ready to face life.

THE BRIDGE BETWEEN FETUS AND BABY

In recent years a great deal has been learned about the physical care of babies, and there are now perinatal and neonatal pediatricians who specialize in this time of life; there are even neonatal physiologists and biochemists. At the Thirteenth International Congress of Paediatrics I attended in Vienna there was a whole section on perinatology that included a series of papers on the influence of birth on tissue function. Dr. Sereni of Milan summarized the worldwide work on how the fetus absorbs and uses his protein, carbohydrate, and fats, and on differences between the biochemistry of the fetus and that of the baby, and the changes that occur in enzyme activity at birth. For instance, the fetus manufactures and stores glycogen in its last weeks in the uterus and breaks it down rapidly after birth to provide glucose; the fetus stores fat before birth and rapidly increases fatty acid breakdown soon after birth. Birth seems to stir the body to activate the enzymes that increase the use of RNA and DNA and enable the body to make protein and nucleic acids, which seem to help in the rapid adjustment of the liver to extrauterine life. Experts at the conference told us how the intestine develops from its immature state at birth, when it is geared to digest milk and not meat and starch, to the stage when it can cope with all foods many months later.

The enzyme lactase, necessary to digest milk, is present in every race at birth, yet in some it seems to disappear as soon as the early milk-drinking stage is over. The baby can also absorb cane sugar, because it has some of the enzyme sucrase but not much amylase, the enzyme needed for starch digestion. I get very exasperated with the sophisticates and moderns who try to push cereal and sieved meat with teaspoons into babies a few weeks old who want only to suck milk and are equipped to do just that. Their kidneys, too, are ready only for nature's first food, human milk. Before birth not much blood flows through the kidneys, but with the change in circulation the flow greatly increases. New enzymes come into action, but it is some time before the kidney can cope efficiently with a higher concentration of minerals than is in human milk—yet there are people who want to feed undiluted cow's milk to babies. Such ignoring of physiology cannot be expected to do any good, yet it continues in the face of scientific evidence that is being produced by research workers at such a rate that the mind boggles.

EMOTIONAL FACTORS

What harm may we be doing to the emotional development of children at birth when we know so little about personality development and the effect on it of birth? There is increasing concern among child psychiatrists at the poor mothering some children receive, and at the increase of behavior problems in children. Rocking, head banging, and sleep disturbances are commoner in babies than they used to be.

In twenty-five years of pediatric practice, mainly concerned with young children and babies, I have seen a change in the problems coming to me. Mothers seem more harassed and confused, and more babies seem to refuse to conform to the picture their parents have of the desirable child.

Is the natural bond between mother and child being disturbed at the very beginning by maternity hospital experiences such as separation at birth and lack of early physical contact between them? Psychiatrists have suggested that depression in the mother may be partly a result of separation. From animal studies we know that separating animals from their mothers at birth has a detrimental effect, even a catastrophic one. Anesthetize a sheep in childbirth and she rejects the lamb. Take a kid away from its mother even for half an hour at birth and she refuses to have it back or let it suckle. Rats will not care for their young well if separated for a time at birth; they cease to bother to retrieve them when they wander off. My Siamese cat is an excellent mother. As each kitten is born she licks it thoroughly all over, and soon it is on the nipple. She leaves her babies for very short periods at first and constantly cleans them. The second day she demands a clean lining for the basket, or she gently carries the kittens off to another place. If she can care for them for two months they are much more attractive, affectionate, and better-house-trained cats than if I give them away at one month.

Mothering

Now there is more awareness among authorities in child care of the needs of the mother and of the fact that bearing a child only makes a woman physically a mother: She has to become a mother emotionally. To achieve this, successful interaction has to occur between the woman and her child, and it can occur quite unrelated to the act of giving birth, as many women who have adopted children can prove; but these are women who want to be mothers emotionally. What of the woman who says, "I am not the motherly type"? Maybe the birth management can influence this. An expert in stud Herefords once told me that when he got a good mother he kept her and all her female offspring, and when he got a bad mother he sent her to the butcher because her calves would be bad mothers too. Maybe the human equivalent of this is to send her back to work and let someone else care for the babies. Mothering is an art that has to be learned, and our management of the maternity hospital may be affecting the normal learning process of the mother. I do think mothering can be taught.

But what of the baby's view of life? Let us consider the fascinating work of Lorenz on imprinting, on the geese that became attached to humans because a human was the first person they saw; and then the work that showed that if the gosling first saw a small red triangle he became correctly imprinted and could attach to other geese. Harlow has shown that the monkey reared artificially cannot relate to its own kind satisfactorily, and that mating and rearing of the young are disturbed. We certainly have some Harlow monkey mothers, but have we also some Harlow monkey children who demonstrate their problems in relating even as small babies? Is it important what they see when first born? Is it important what handling they get? It has been shown that if the puppy and kitten are not stimulated in the genital area in that first good cleanup, and if they are not well licked very soon after birth, they may not even survive.

The Baby's Needs

Obviously we cannot draw direct conclusions from the handling required by animals, but it is reasonable to assume that there are some basic needs for newborn babies. It is also perhaps reasonable to assume that they relate to the physical needs we have already discussed. Why is the baby so acutely sensitive to changes of position; why is he born with a startle reflex, a rooting reflex, and a tonic neck reflex and a sucking reflex—all of which disappear or greatly decrease in the first few months? Why is he so sensitive to skin touch, and why do most mothers long to hold their babies and get them to the breast very soon after delivery? His vision is poor at birth, so it is unlikely that anything as clear as a shape has to be seen, but there is a suggestion that the oval of a face is significant.

Why do babies love rhythmical movement? It is easily demonstrated that a baby is more easily quieted when crying by nursing it over the heart and rocking. What strange cultural movement took rocking chairs and cradles from Anglo-Saxon women and gave them an obsession about spoiling children? This disease did not afflict the Mediterranean people or much of Europe. Perhaps it was part of the cold austere Calvinistic doctrine. I find myself constantly telling mothers that it is not possible to spoil a baby by giving it too much love and security; but my idea of love and security, which I think is also the baby's, is not always the mother's. A spotlessly clean, elaborately dressed baby being cuddled and kissed can be a very unhappy, uncomfortable baby, getting indigestion from its artificial food and being left to cry for its four-hourly feed.

Love and security to a baby mean having his physical needs met, food that he can enjoy and keep down, relaxed sleep, reasonably prompt attention to his call for help when he is wet and in an uncomfortable position, or cold or hot. Illingworth says that the more relaxed and calm the routine and the more patient the mother, the more likely her child is to sleep. Is the rocking New York infant craving for the rocking and close physical contact it missed as a tiny baby? Is the autistic uncommunicating child, rocking and fascinated with machinery and moving wheels, somehow a particular type of child who has withdrawn early from the kind of human contact he was offered at birth and in the maternity hospital and by our infant-care practices?

My early rebellion against traditional baby-care teaching arose from my own instinctive feeling that what I was being asked to do was wrong, in the sense that it was not what my baby wanted or what I wanted. Yet my Calvinistic upbringing also taught me that I had to acquire self-discipline and a sense of responsibility. Not that I ever acquired a high degree of self-discipline, because I react emotionally to every situation; but the ideal is somewhere in the middle. Both mother and child do have instinctive responses to each other and the process of reaching maturity involves gaining responsible control over oneself and one's environment.

Thirty years ago Margaret Ribble wrote her book *The Rights of Infants*, the result of many years spent observing mothers and children in "an attempt to discover how the satisfaction of the psychological needs of small infants might contribute to the enrichment and stability of emotional life and to our human capacities to live, learn and adjust more happily." The book is a classic to which very little of significance has been added, despite an enormous volume of research in the field. She emphasizes the fact that mother and baby are still a functional unit, and that separation threatens the life of the infant until after he can speak and move about. She opposes the idea that you spoil a baby by nursing and feeding and attending to his cries, and points out his sensitivity to touch, pressure, warmth, and being moved about, and his pleasure in nursing, his acute sense of smell and position. These feelings and senses are present at birth, and it seems to me that the surest way to spoil a child is to fail to meet his needs. His biological needs will be very close to his psychological ones.

The washing or oiling all over after birth is more than a cleaning process: It provides skin stimulation in the most sensitive areas of face (particularly mouth, nose, forehead) and genitalia. Movement of arms and legs stimulates breathing reflexes, as does skin stimulation.

The baby in the uterus is accustomed to the movement of the mother's body. It must seem strange when it all stops and he is no longer held warm and secure and rocked as she moves. Admittedly he is upside down while in the uterus, but at least we should not think that rocking and holding him firmly wrapped in mother's arms could spoil him. Rather they are a way of gradually accustoming him to his stationary crib. Dr. Ribble suggests that if more mothers met their babies' need for rhythmical movement in the early months there would be less need for pacifiers and other sucking activity that the child adopts in response to his need for rhythmical movement.

THE IMPORTANCE OF PHYSICAL CONTACT

Yarrow, studying the correlations between infant development and maternal care, found that the maternal actions that correlated best with good infant progress were (a) the extent to which the mother provided conditions that facilitated learning by encouragement and materials, (b) the appropriateness of the materials and stimulation to the development of the child, (c) social stimulation, and (d) the *amount of physical contact*.

Surely all these must be encouraged in the hospital, and the modern, sophisticated mother guided to meet her baby's needs. So often mothers tell me that their babies were so "good" in the hospital but cried a lot as soon as they got home. Was being "good" lying quiet and satisfied with the stimulation of a daily bath by expert hands and four-hourly feeds added to if he was still hungry? Or was the mother not told the truth? Or could she not yet recognize the cry of her baby, separated from her in the nursery? Or had her milk supply suddenly fallen in going home and had her inexperience in meeting the baby's needs been the reason why he had now become "bad"? It is in most cases the last, and it should be a function of the maternity hospital staff to make sure that every mother has had an opportunity in the hospital to care for her own baby and understand its needs. It is only too easy for well-trained, experienced staff to keep a baby contented while in the hospital, and the inexperienced mother may well wonder what has happened when the transformation occurs on going home.

How then does the woman rate who artificially feeds her baby, who props up the bottle or uses one of those monstrous insults to any infant—an artificial bottle-holder on a stand—and nurses the baby as little as possible? A maternity hospital can provide all the biological needs, but not always in the best way. Only too often the baby is taken away at birth by a nurse, has the mucus sucked out, is given oxygen, wrapped up warmly in a crib, perhaps in metallic paper or on an electric blanket, put in an air-conditioned or warmed room away from the mother, and given a bottle of water or glucose to suck, with the mother being given barely a glimpse, and often not a touch for the first two days.

Is there any real reason why the mother should not take an active part in meeting the baby's early needs? Many doctors say she should, and if Yarrow is right in saying that his work shows that the child's ability to cope with stress can be related to the mother's ability to adapt the environment to the child's needs early in life, then the mother needs closer contact with her baby in the hospital and more instruction in meeting the child's needs. She becomes a mother as she accepts the protective nurturing role and becomes involved to the depths of her being with the helpless little human creature she has borne.

What You Have to Learn

If you thought you were going to lie in bed surrounded by flowers, receiving admiring visitors, writing letters, restoring your hair, face, and fingernails to their former beauty, then let me disillusion you. Even if your husband has remembered the flowers and put the birth notice in the paper (which he may well have overlooked) there is a lot to do in the hospital. You are now a woman of responsibilities with a baby to feed and a lot to learn. Even if you are a triple-certificate nurse and know all about babies, it is quite different with your own, and you are learning to feel and meet his particular needs. No grim determination to bring up a model baby, please! No saying that he has to fit into your way of life and get trained early! The vast majority of women find that bearing a child arouses strong emotion, and they find themselves overwhelmed with a tremendous desire to give the child the best care possible. Unfortunately many measure this in terms of money and material goods or cleanliness and asepsis. I see beautiful baby clothes and very expensive equipment that looks more like keeping up with the Joneses than meeting baby's real needs, and I've seen some very clean unhappy babies.

So let's have a look at him as he lies in his crib. There is really no need to be afraid for him. He has a strong desire to survive and nature who prepared him so well for the strenuous experience of birth has allowed for some very uncertain handling by inexperienced mothers. There will be many a time when you will prod him to make sure he is breathing, and you will find that not only do your senses become much more acute to his needs but you become aware of silence and automatically investigate it—usually unnecessary for the baby but good training for minding a two-year-old when silence always means trouble, even if it's only your lipstick all over the wallpaper.

For that first couple of days both you and your baby will be glad to rest, and even if you have a crib beside your bed during the day it is best to have him in the nursery at night and while visitors are with you. His resistance to infection is not good, and it is not fair to let all the visitors go all over him; through glass will do for everyone except father, who had better find out what it feels like to hold his own baby.

FEEDING

It is essential that with your first baby you have some instruction in managing the first feeds. Unless you are familiar with the technique of breast-feeding from watching others, you will not know how, for this is an art to be learned. You may think you will know how, but somehow you will find yourself being very awkward, and if baby chews around and does not get onto the nipple properly your nipples soon get sore; then he gets mad and refuses to go on—and you feel rejected and dissolve in tears. So let's get it right from the first.

Baby has a very strong instinct to get food. Touch his cheek, and he turns toward you and his mouth starts to move. His little tongue curls up at the sides into a deep channel and he starts to suck. He wants the nipple planted firmly, well into his mouth, so that he can clamp down on the areola with his gums and put pressure on the lacteal sinuses and force milk out. The best position for him will be cradled in your arm, face against bare breast. Guide the nipple into his mouth, and hold your breast between index and second finger so that you support it and prevent its pulling out of his mouth. Never push him on by the back of the head; he automatically resists and pulls back. These first feeds are very short, just a minute or two; there is only a little colostrum to get, so they are practice feeds for you both, and he must not suck at an empty breast and hurt the nipples. After a minute or two, press on his chin or the sides of his cheeks and make him let go; don't pull him off. Many babies at first do not suck well; they are tired from labor. So don't be impatient and don't be too disappointed if he is kept in the crib for a couple of days, because this is common hospital practice. Ideally he should be fed when he wants to be, but this is very difficult for you to recognize with your first baby. The usual routine is to feed him five or six times a day (i.e., about every four hours), starting about 5:00 A.M. and with none after midnight while you are in the hospital, to let you have your rest—though some hospitals will allow the baby to be brought to you if you ask.

When the breasts fill on the third day, you may be very uncomfortable, particularly if the milk came in during the night, and it is best to let the nurses know as soon as you realize your breasts are hardening so that baby can be brought in to relieve them. However, he may find it hard to grip on, and some women get such tight breasts that it may be necessary to hand-express the milk.

Most mothers and babies have some minor adjustment problems at this stage, because we do not manage the first two days as nature intended, with many short sucking periods to accustom the baby to sucking and opening up the ducts. However, this stage soon passes. During the time in the hospital you must learn the best positions for feeding, with baby at an angle of about 45 degrees.

THE SUCKLING REFLEXES

Successful lactation depends on the establishment of the suckling reflexes—the let-down reflex and the secretory reflex. The first occurs when a nervous impulse passes from the nipple to the hypothalamus in the brain, and from there to the posterior

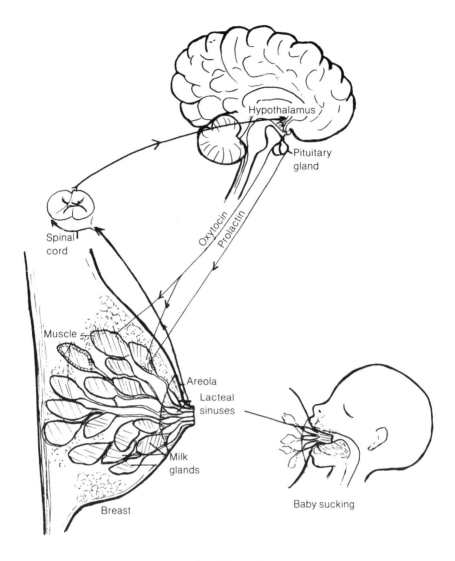

Suckling reflexes

pituitary gland, which releases oxytocin; this hormone then passes by the bloodstream to the muscle tissue surrounding the glands in the breast and forces milk down into the ducts and lacteal sinuses where the baby can get it. The secretory reflex involves stimulation from the nipple again, going up to the hypothalamus, but from there it passes to the anterior pituitary gland, which releases a different hormone. This one is prolactin, which stimulates milk secretion and in animals can be shown to produce mothering behavior; it passes down to the glands and stimulates them to produce milk.

It takes time to get these reflexes well established in the first lactation, and it is a few weeks before you get the feeling of milk coming down into the breast, though you know it has come by seeing it drip from the opposite side when the baby is sucking. It may come too fast at first and baby may gulp, or if you are nervous you may secrete another hormone, adrenalin, which tends to delay the milk and prevent it from coming down properly. Obviously, if you have unsympathetic staff or nurses who do not understand the technique of breast-feeding or who give contradictory instructions, you may be very confused and get off to a bad start.

LEARNING TO BREAST-FEED

I must admit that most maternity hospitals do not seem to teach breast-feeding well. It seems to me that some very rigid old-fashioned methods are still being taught, and there is no surer way to make lactation fail than to insist on strict four-hourly feeds, with no night feed, and to make feeds ten minutes each side. The ten-minute-each-side rule is probably the worst, for ten minutes may be too long and cause the baby to suck on an empty breast and hurt the nipple. A much better way is to allow the baby to

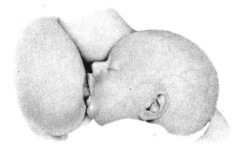
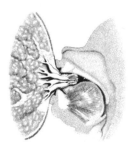

The proper position of the infant's mouth on the breast

suck on one side for about five minutes, or until he eases off, then change to the other side for about five minutes—or when he pulls away—then back to the first. This way he does not suck for so long on either nipple without resting it, and if the mother makes sure that there is some milk there when he first starts he is unlikely to suck at an empty breast.

Breast-feeding can be an enjoyable experience, but it takes time; so learn all you can and don't fuss. Baby may even need a little extra artificial feed at a couple of the nursings first, though three-hourly feeding for a few days can overcome this quite often.

WIND

Babies often swallow air while feeding, particularly if they are allowed to lie horizontal and are not properly elevated. The best way to get the air up is to hold the baby upright against your body and pat his tail to vibrate him so that he burps. Some people prefer rubbing his back; I find that this often brings up the milk as well. You can certainly learn this technique in the hospital, but don't work too hard at it. If there is no result in a few minutes, lay baby down for five minutes; when you pick him up you usually have success. There is often wind after the first breast and none after the second.

HANDLING

Baby is very sensitive to changes in position and very sensitive to touch; he hates sudden movement and sudden noise, so gentle, confident handling is indicated. The skin stimulation in wiping him as you change his diaper and wash him is probably important, and he likes to be wrapped up warmly and firmly after changing, as though he were back in the security of the womb.

You will bathe him yourself after watching a demonstration bath, and a slippery little eel you will find him; but the nurse will show you a good grip and there is no need to feel nervous.

Get as much experience as you can in the hospital in handling, changing, bathing, and feeding the baby. This is your chance to do it all under supervision and to gain confidence. I am sure that many of the blasé women we meet these days who say that they don't want to breast-feed, and who say they are not going to be tied down to a baby, are merely very insecure, and have great trouble adjusting to their female role, preferring not to try rather than to fail, and passing it all off as sophistication. I am sure that our maternity hospitals are failing these women very badly in not providing adequate teaching and encouragement; there is no need for women to breast-feed if they feel repelled by it, but most are willing and anxious to learn more about their baby's needs and how to satisfy them.

Some Special Babies

THE LOW-BIRTH-WEIGHT BABY

Babies that weigh under five and a half pounds at birth constitute about 7 percent of all births. Most of them are babies born prematurely, but some are babies that have not thrived in the uterus. Of the latter some have failed to thrive because of the mother's ill health (e.g., high blood pressure or kidney trouble) and others may have been ill while in the uterus, they may have a congenital abnormality, or just have had a very small placenta, which restricted their food intake. The small-for-date or dysmature baby, as we call him, needs to be watched carefully even if he is actually on term, because in such babies blood sugar tends to fall, and they may need to have blood samples examined at intervals. They are always given extra sugar and they usually thrive and give less trouble than the bigger baby that was more premature.

The premature baby is not ready for individual existence and when he is born he will have more problems than other babies in adapting all systems from his parasitic existence to his individual existence. The first difficulty will be with breathing and this is a vital one. He will be more upset than the full-term baby by any drugs the mother has had during labor; there is more likely to be fluid still in his chest; and the ribs are still soft and it will be harder for him to take his first breath because his lungs are immature. He is also accustomed to a very moist atmosphere and was meant to stay there a bit longer; so he often has to go into a humidicrib with high humidity (90 percent), and extra oxygen at body temperature, and alarm gadgets that ring bells if he stops breathing so that he gets very prompt attention. The doctor may hasten his delivery a little by lifting his head out with forceps and performing an episiotomy to save any delay and pressure on his head; and if the mother needs an anesthetic, it will be a local. He will get cold very easily, partly because his temperature-regulating mechanism is not ready for the outside world, but also because he has not had time to get a good layer of fat under his skin. He will appear to be a very scraggy little mortal, about the size of a skinned rabbit and not unlike one. His skin looks transparent and the blood vessels show through; his ears and skull bones are soft because the cartilage and bone are not well formed, most of the calcium being deposited in bone in the last two months. A warmed crib or the warm humidicrib is essential.

The premature baby is not ready to drink, and even if he is willing to suck he tires so easily that he is usually fed through a little transparent polythene tube put through his nose and down his stomach and left there for up to three days at a time. This tube-feeding is a wonderful asset because small quantities can be given often, and with it the baby is less likely to vomit and get the milk in his lungs. It is usual to feed premature babies within six hours of birth, just with glucose and water, and then to progress to milk—breast milk if possible, because it is more easily digested. The small baby needs breast milk because his resistance to infection is poor, his stomach is not ready to cope with anything but the simplest food, he needs the extra iron in breast milk since he will not absorb it as a mixture, and he thrives better on breast milk.

This will mean that the mother has to express milk, and feeding a breast pump is not a great emotional experience; in fact, many women faced with a baby staying in the hospital for a few weeks refuse even to try to produce milk. In most hospitals breast milk is the standard nourishment for premature babies, even if their mothers have none. Some mothers have too much and an effort is made to keep a milk bank going. I remember finding the nurse in charge of the ward at one maternity hospital very indignant one morning when I arrived. "That Mrs. S.," she said, "is refusing to express her milk and asked me why I could not use pooled breast milk for the baby." It really is surprising what some women expect to have done for them.

Expressing their milk makes most mothers feel better about that unpleasant experience of going home without a baby: At least the mother is doing something for her baby that no one else can do, in spite of all that medical-scientific equipment surrounding him. Do you know that a humidicrib costs as much as a small car?

There have been great strides in the care of the premature baby in recent years, and now with oxygen analyzers to measure how much oxygen he is breathing, and blood glucose tests to make sure his brain is getting the glucose it needs, and very superior methods of keeping his body temperature regulated, he is less likely to suffer permanent ill effects from his early arrival.

The commonest complications are breathing difficulties, jaundice, and infection. The jaundice used to cause brain damage before the days of exchange transfusions, but now the level of pigment can be measured and when it reaches a dangerous height an exchange transfusion can be done. To prevent infection, the baby is nursed in a special room with special precautions against infection. While he is in the special ward it is important that you go to visit him. You may feel a bit silly visiting a baby that is oblivious of your existence, but you need to see and touch him to know he is your baby, or almost grieve as if you had lost him; and that is no way to get ready for bringing him home.

Depending on how early he was, there are some hazards during the first year. Most premature babies get anemic and need an iron mixture from about six weeks. They are prone to infection, particularly chest infection, and should be kept away from people with coughs, colds, and skin infections.

The premature baby is not ready for all the stimulation of the outside world, and should not be handled by visitors and excited. He may well tend to be overexcitable as a result of the early birth, anyway; but for the first few weeks he may be very quiet, and of course he will not smile or respond as early as the full-term baby. His age is measured from conception, not birth really, but most premature babies seem to have just about caught up by twelve months. As he loses heat easily, you may be told not to bathe him; just oil him for the first week or so, or else sponge him every second day and then progress to bathing every few days.

As a rough guide, you will get your baby home just about when he was normally due, and he will not gain weight as fast as if he had stayed in the uterus. You will get him when he is over five and a half pounds, all being well.

There may be some feeding difficulties, since he has been tube-fed and then learned to suck a bottle. You will be asked to come into the hospital for a few days, or at least to come in daily and get him used to the breast.

The premature baby usually catches up in general growth with the full-term, but some of the very tiny ones stay smaller than average, and some of the small-for-date babies who did not have sufficient food while in the uterus in their very vital growing stage do not catch up in general size. Studies of intelligence show in general that the premature baby's brain develops satisfactorily, but that he has more reading difficulties and some learning difficulties even though he has normal intelligence. It is thought that this may be due to the unusual experience of the first months of life, but it is just as well to know that he may need some extra help when he starts school.

THE BABY WHO HAS HAD A DIFFICULT BIRTH

Instrumental delivery, breech birth, and Caesarean section babies have all had some difficulty adjusting to their individual existence. This often means that they go for a few days to a special ward where their mothers can see and touch them but not have much more access.

The instruments often make a pressure mark on the sides of the head, but that soon goes away. They do not harm the child; rather they have in some cases saved his life. Such a baby is likely to have more head molding and you may think he has a funny elongated head, but that soon gets back to normal, too. The breech and Caesarean babies have no molding and look rather more presentable than the others for the first few days.

All these babies often have what we call mild cerebral irritation, rather like concussion. There is no permanent harm, but they tend to vomit, the heart rate and breathing may speed up, and their body temperature may vary more than normal, and some may be irritable with a little high-pitched or grunting cry.

Some too, will be more liable to jaundice and also may have some tiny hemorrhages from pressure. These are rather like little flea bites on the face as a rule, but you may see small patches of blood in the whites of the eyes; they will go away in due course and cause no trouble.

By the time you take the baby home most of his symptoms will have settled, but he may be irritable and it may be advisable not to bathe him every day. You should visit the baby clinic nurse or your doctor to make sure all is going well, because with your first you do not know what to expect, and I have often found mothers quite unnecessarily putting up with a very unhappy baby until their postnatal check at six weeks. Caesarean babies are also liable to anemia and may need iron mixture.

TWINS

Twins come in two different types. Uniovular come from one ovum that has split. They are identical, and of the same sex, share their outer membrane, and have one placenta. Binovular twins come from two ova, can be of different sexes, have a complete set of membranes, and their own placenta—but the placentas can be so close together that they are often thought to be one.

There is more risk to the twin who is born second, since he has to go through two labors; but the outlook for twins is very good if the mother has had prenatal care and they have been diagnosed. Twin babies tend to be smaller than average and the mother tends to come into labor a few weeks early so this may mean a few days in the intensive care ward for the babies. It is best to take both home together if possible.

Many women can breast-feed twins, and the usual pattern is to feed both first thing in the morning at the breast and then to alternate breast and bottle for the rest of the day; but some mothers manage to fully breast-feed for the first few weeks.

Twins tend to get anemic, particularly if not breast-fed, so an iron mixture is usually given to them at about six weeks. Managing twins is really a full-time job, particularly when they are both crying at once; but I am sure nature gives twins good mothers—they all seem to manage very well. It is important to treat them as individuals: Don't dress them the same except for fun sometimes, and don't worry if one needs more nursing than the other. You cannot treat all children in the same way; they must be treated according to their needs, but twins do get jealous. It must be very trying to have to compete all the time for attention, but then a twin provides company, too; so look at the whole situation from the babies' point of view.

9

The First Weeks
Home

Most mothers will be taking the baby home about the fourth day after birth. I often wonder as I watch the new family leaving the hospital if they know what is in store: mother happy and slim again (what a wonderful feeling to be in one's normal clothes!), a nurse carrying the baby, his first appearance in his own lovingly prepared layette; proud father with car at the door, bassinet ready, feeling very aware of his new responsibilities. Mothers of first babies are always anxious to get out of the hospital as soon as possible. The mother longs to have her baby and her husband to herself and revel in her newfound maturity as mother and wife. But often it is more practical to stay a few days longer and make sure she is really on her feet and her lactation off to a good start. Certainly if she goes home before the seventh day she needs some domestic help or she may lose both her milk and her morale.

Every people has its traditional taboos and rites for mothers of new babies that guard them from the herd for a little while. Even a generation ago it was accepted that a maiden aunt or mother-in-law would come and stay with the young mother, or she would go to mom for a few days. Now, as often as not, the new father takes his vacation and the new mother comes home to a house where he has been alone for a week, with usually not even a community nurse to call and with no domestic help. In the hospital she had all her meals brought to her, the dirty dishes whisked away; the soiled diapers vanished to the laundry; the crib was already made up with clean linen when she went to put baby down; there were clean clothes ready for him after the bath; if she felt a bit tired, a nurse did the bath for her; her room was swept, her bed was made, her flowers were given water, and as likely as not she had a rest period that was not to be disturbed. If baby cried or looked queer to her inexperienced eye, her call for help was promptly attended to; she sat down or lay down whenever she felt like it.

It is good to be home, but has father ever got the meals, done the housework, or washed a diaper, or even done the grocery shopping? The spirit may be willing, but he, too, has preconceived ideas about the joys of fatherhood that may not include such earthy realities. Let's hope you gave him a shopping list before you left the hospital: ice cream in the freezer, a good stock of chops, bread and butter, potatoes, fruit, frozen vegetables, eggs, breakfast cereal—but then you know what you eat and he may as well find out what food costs! If you have not already got baby's needs, then a bottle and nipples is the first essential (your milk supply may drop when you go home and a little extra may be needed), and orange juice or rose hip syrup will start at three weeks. You'll also need talc, cotton balls, baby soap, safety pins, baby oil, methylated alcohol, and a soothing cream for his tail, such as zinc and castor oil, in case he gets chafed.

If you can have a woman about the house for a few days it really is worthwhile. Perhaps the new maternal grandmother can come—you may not be quite up to supervision by the new paternal grandmother—just to enable you to stay in bed a little longer and have breakfast and doze off again. Don't imagine that when the obstetrician cheerfully discharged you, and told you to see him when baby was six weeks old, it meant that there would be no problems. Perhaps no problems to worry a specialist gynecologist, but the time after returning home is not an easy, untroubled period, and it is a very important one. For every woman it is a time when she needs encouragement and some company, but not numerous visitors. Most of the problems of the first weeks are easily overcome with some planning and an acceptance of the fact that this is not the time for independence.

Getting Back to Normal

It takes six weeks for the uterus to return to normal size and for the relaxed ligaments of the pelvis to tighten up and carry the body weight for long periods in comfort; tummy muscles, pelvic floor muscles, and perineal muscles have to regain their tone. You may feel that everything is dropping out if you stay on your feet for long, and that feeling may be more noticeable with the second baby than with the first. Most hospitals provide a physiotherapy service while you are resident, and these cheerful, healthy girls put your protesting muscles through their paces; but that is not enough—you must keep the exercises up after you go home. Every time you think of it, tighten up your tummy muscles and your perineum. The knee-chest exercise is not advised at this period, since it is thought risky if people have blood clots and air has been known to get into veins. Backache is common after childbirth and it is relieved by short rests, by special exercises, or most of all by a firm foundation garment. Some physiotherapists may tell you that you must rely on tightening up your muscles and holding yourself together to get back to normal, and that will happen in due course as you work at it; but in the meantime get a girdle and be held together in comfort. One can improve on Nature but one must not defy her! Avoid anything tight around the legs (garters or tight legs in the panty girdle), because this could cause pressure on varicose veins. Avoid standing for long periods, because this delays the emptying of veins in the pelvic area and legs. The veins in the lower abdomen and legs have been subjected to pressure from the uterus during pregnancy, and they are often dilated, and end up as varicose veins and hemorrhoids (piles), which can be uncomfortable. Backache will be made worse by incorrect methods of lifting. Doing postnatal exercises conscientiously will hasten the return of your figure to normal and this is important. As Lord Peter Wimsey said of his firstborn, who had caused his wife, Harriet, some trouble, "It's a very interesting addition to you, darling, but it'd be a damn poor substitute." A husband usually reacts favorably to seeing the mother giving tender loving care (TLC) to his offspring, but he still wants the woman he married. You may also need some attention to your hair and wardrobe.

This is no time to act tough physically and resume full duties; nor is it time to move or to have renovations done; and it is no time to be caring for a sick or elderly relative. You need some TLC too, and you need rest periods, sleep, good food, and hygiene.

Avoid constipation; it puts pressure on the hemorrhoids. Strong laxatives may make matters worse and cause a clot in the hemorrhoid (thrombosed pile), and that is agony. The best is a high-roughage diet: prunes, bran, whole wheat bread and, to stimulate the bowel wall, fruit and plenty to drink; but a fecal softener may be advisable. There may also be a recurrence of vaginal bleeding at this time owing to the extra activity. It goes away with rest.

The Household Chores

Simplify the housework, close your eyes to some of the dust. House-proud mothers may be good housekeepers, but they are not very comfortable people to live with. Plan simple meals that will not be ruined if baby demands dinner just as father is about to be served. A few casseroles made ahead and some "take-out" chicken brought home by father can go a long way to solving that problem temporarily. Breast-feeding baby will require some extra attention to diet, for a balanced diet is needed to keep both mother and baby well. Calcium from milk and cheese; vitamins B and C from whole-grain cereal, fresh vegetables, and fruit; iron and protein from meat, particularly liver and kidney—all are important. Many women find drinking two pints of milk a day rather an unpleasant way to get the calcium, but this can be chocolate drink or café au lait, ice cream, yogurt, cheese, and even a calcium tablet if you are off dairy products and on a polyunsaturated jag; but yogurt at least seems to be favored by the cardiologists.

The laundry is a real chore, particularly if this is the second baby and there is a lot of toddler's washing too. Diaper-washing services are reliable and very satisfactory and can be a real boon in the first weeks after leaving the hospital at least. Disposable diapers would be great if they were less expensive and really were disposable; but they do not go down toilets, the garbage man may refuse to take them, and they do not burn very well. However, disposable diapers can save a lot of laundry time. If the diaper service is too expensive you'll just have to wash the diapers yourself and dry them in the sun or in a drier. The whole laundry situation will amaze and overwhelm you until you get organized with soaking buckets, daily washing, and a routine. If someone can do the main washing and ironing for you for the first weeks it does help; you will feel much less tired. If you have to iron, at least only do the essential things and do the ironing sitting down. Accept any generous neighbor's offer to hang out washing or to take the toddler for a walk.

Coming home after the second confinement may be more tiring than after the first, because the two-year-old thinks you are still at her disposal and she has missed you. Suddenly you have to adjust to being the mother of two, less mobile and more dependent on others; yet everyone expects you to manage better with your second child and you get less attention. If a neighbor brings you a cake or an apple pie, you will feel incredibly grateful and regard her as a friend for life. Don't ruin the effect of her kind deed by trying to repay her at once. So many independent modern girls find it hard to accept kind gestures graciously. I always found it a problem.

The Emotional Adjustment

The psychological adjustment to becoming a twenty-four-hour-a-day mother is quite considerable, and this is associated with hormone changes in the first weeks of the childbirth that will confuse you. The whole endocrine system has to return to normal balance. Removal of the placenta with its hormone secretions, the establishment of lactation with secretion of prolactin and oxytocin, the adjustment of the hypothalamus and pituitary, all have emotional accompaniments and exaggerate your normal reactions. Joy and tears are very close together; you may be lying back feeding your baby, completely relaxed, ecstatically gazing at his beauty, and a short half hour later crying over a pile of dirty diapers and a burned milk saucepan, feeling too tired to cope. If you are alone you will find this emotional instability very hard to live with, and you may even doubt your sanity.

You may have had those "third- or fifth-day blues" in the

hospital—about 50 percent of women do. It is a weak, weepy, depressed, apathetic, letdown kind of feeling; it certainly has a reactive element in it: After nine months of waiting for the new and possibly dreaded experience of labor, once it is successfully surmounted there is bound to be some reaction. It is commoner in women who are confined in a hospital, and may also be aggravated by drugs; sleeping tablets are often ordered for a few nights after the birth and can lead to variable reactions in some women. In general, it is best to avoid drugs or keep their use to a minimum and just have a pain-reliever if the hemorrhoids or the episiotomy sutures or the headache after the epidural block are too painful. Keeping the baby nearby, instead of in the hospital nursery, may reduce the reaction, but it can make matters worse if the nurses are not readily available and the mother is too much alone. It is quite normal to be apprehensive and to need help and supervision.

About 10 percent of women experience marked depression after leaving the hospital. Some psychiatrists suggest that this may be due to separation of mother and baby in the hospital, and they recommend that the best treatment for the mild depression that follows is to make sure the mother can devote her time to the baby and have someone with her to do the housework and cooking. The depression may be more severe in the controlled and in-dependent woman, and in the woman who has cherished a glamorous and unrealistic concept of motherhood. The less she is aware that babies are very demanding, have different sleep patterns from other humans, cry and vomit, in fact are completely irresponsible at both ends, the more likely she is to be depressed and feel inadequate. Fatigue is inevitable; nature makes sure that a woman feels tired to ensure that she gets rest, because if she does not rest she surely loses her milk.

Emotional reactions are variable. A good cry now and again is a great relief; and in a few weeks you are back on an even keel, though far from having your prepregnancy poise. You may find that you are nervous driving the car. That is a very common reaction and it may be best not to drive for a few weeks. Don't bottle up your fears and worries; go and talk to a friend or the doctor or the pediatric nurse. I have had weeping mothers tell me that they could not trust themselves to be alone with the baby;

they were terrified that they would hurt it, even throw it out the window, and they were horrified that the thought even entered their heads. I think that most mothers do at times have these frightening thoughts, and I sometimes wonder if this is nature's way of making mothers realize how very helpless a newborn baby is. But it is more probably the mother's reaction to feeling trapped, tied down, and perhaps inadequate to meet the child's needs.

We can learn a great deal from birds and animals, by just watching nature's methods of insuring survival in other species. I never cease to be fascinated with the conscientious mothering that my Siamese cat gives to even her most unattractive illegitimate offspring, the preparation for confinement as she explores my wardrobe and study, finally choosing for the last litter some of my precious reprints and references for this book. Then the feeding, grooming, protecting, and instructing in hygiene and foraging that goes on puts many a human mother to shame. Cows have their problems, too. The boss cow of our little herd is a huge Hereford we know as Spotty Face; she leads the way to pasture and water, she pushes others off the juicy grass, but she is having real problems with junior—a smart little bull calf who sees no reason to be washed or to come when mother calls and dashes off in the opposite direction while his anxious mother searches in the long grass making motherly noises.

There is no doubt, as Robertson has observed in *Determinants of Infant Behaviour,* that adequate mothering in all mammals is associated with a considerable increase in anxiety during the time of caring for the young. Good mothers are anxious about the welfare of their babies, and it really does annoy me to hear a doctor, nurse, or schoolteacher refer disparagingly to "anxious mothers" as if they were abnormal.

I am sure that nearly all mothers want their babies looked after well, even if they themselves do not want to do the day-to-day care. Such women usually feel inadequate and uncertain of their own ability to care for a baby, and they think it is better to do their career job and pay someone else to care for the baby, and they may well be right. The mother with a constantly crying baby or with a child with a chronic illness usually does all she can to help her child, and if her efforts are not successful, she starts to dislike the child and even wants to hurt it. A woman becoming aware of these feelings is shocked and distressed and will often not talk about them; but it is most important that she should get help for the child. As soon as he stops crying, gets over the pain he had in his tummy, and ceases to be a monster and becomes a lovable sleeping baby who smiles when he wakes, the mother finds that she adores him. I mention these feelings to let mothers and fathers know that they are very real in those who get them, that they are not a sign of wickedness or insanity, but a sign that mother and baby need more help from their understanding pediatrician or general practitioner.

The father must be prepared to accept that woman's normal unpredictability and variable moods will be exaggerated in the weeks following childbirth, and this is his chance to be the strong, calm one. But he will not really understand, so it is better for the mother not to wait and pour it all out as soon as he comes home from work; he may just be shocked and confused. After all, he is just getting used to the awful responsibility of having brought a child into the world, and finds he has a temporarily useless wife absorbed in the baby. The suggestion that she is having strange, frightening thoughts may well be the last straw. For some women this is really a disturbing and prolonged episode and they need help quickly. The father should be taught to recognize the symptoms: Persisting depression, excessive fatigue, inability to sleep, and apathy indicate that a doctor must be called and that someone is needed to help with the baby.

Mother-Baby Adjustment

It takes time to get to know baby, and if he has pains in his tummy he will not be very interested in making your acquaintance, apart from uttering loud protesting cries day and night. Many mothers find it quite hard to get really interested in the child until he starts responding; in fact they may feel intensely hurt and rejected if all their efforts to make this tiny scrap of humanity happy are failing; and if he vomits or fights the breast this really appears to be rejecting behavior. The first real mother-baby adjustment is in the feeding situation, and a mother feels very inadequate if a baby does not suck properly or pulls off and screams. This is usually due to an unsatisfactory feeding technique, to lack of understanding of how babies suck and how the milk flows (whether from breast or bottle), or perhaps to unsuitable artificial feeding; cow's-milk allergy is quite common.

All the mother usually needs is to have a feed supervised by someone who knows what it is all about, to check technique and give some expert advice on managing a feed. Even if things went smoothly in the hospital and the baby seemed to have a good grip and to be getting on well and there was plenty of milk, the move away from instant help often leaves the mother anxious; this disturbs her milk let-down, so that it comes down unevenly or intermittently. It really exasperates the baby to get a gush one second and nothing the next; he may well get wind or come off and fight.

A good way to find out what it is like to be a baby is to lie flat on your back and suck all the way through a ten-ounce bottle of milk. It is not easy, and your jaws may ache. At least it will teach you not to prod the poor baby every time he stops sucking to rest his jaws and tongue, an irresistible urge that many mothers seem to have.

Think what it must be like to have the milk gush into your mouth or not come at all. Try to enjoy feed time and don't expect lactation to be firmly established till six weeks after birth. If the mother is not supplying half the milk by then she usually wants to give up; but it may well be worthwhile to complement one or two feedings a day for a few weeks to get baby happy and mother relaxed so that the let-down comes more normally. The first weeks home often mean a drop in milk supply from tension and a cranky baby; that can be corrected. It is really no trouble to have two ounces of formula in a bottle standing in warm water in case it is needed. Baby will probably demand six feeds in twenty-four hours for the first weeks, but if the supply is adequate the number can be reduced to five quite soon by the simple expedient of allowing only a quick suck for comfort at the feed you want to drop. Most mothers find that going to bed early and letting baby decide the time for the night feeds works best. He often wakes about midnight and both mother and baby get more sleep.

Sleep is absolutely essential for everyone—father, mother, and baby—and without it everyone gets cranky and intolerant; so mother must have an afternoon nap if baby is keeping her up at night.

Routine

The above may all sound a bit disorganized and suggest that I am not in favor of routine, but this is not so. It takes a few weeks to get the milk supply regulated and mother and baby used to everyday tasks. Babies love routine; at least, they like to know what is coming next, though they have no idea of time and half an hour either way on the feeds means nothing. It gives security to have order. Of course, if someone wakes the baby with a sudden loud noise, like the telephone or doorbell, he assumes that he has been awakened for something. Food is uppermost in the infant's mind, so as often as not he begins sucking and nuzzling. He can, however, usually be soothed by rocking and singing.

It is a pity that the lullaby is so often ignored by the modern mother. I have know a mother to buy a record of lullabies to put on for the baby—an idea almost as extraordinary as that little pulsating gadget to put under the baby's pillow to sound like the mother's heart! Let's be reasonable about this business of relating to a baby. A short time ago he was tucked up in his mother's uterus, held warm and tight and secure surrounded by the sounds of surging blood as it pulsated around her body, and hearing the lub-dub of her beating heart, and constantly being rocked as she went about her daily work. Is it reasonable to expect him to enjoy a silent, still crib and even to keep himself warm in it? All babies hate sudden noises, but most love car engines and vacuum cleaners, except just when they start, and they all love rhythmic rocking and being fondled and held against their mother's body; they hear her heartbeat again and as she hums a lullaby they feel the vibration as well as hearing a soothing sound. Don't think that a mother has to be a prima donna to satisfy an infant, and he has no need for the words or even the right tune; so don't be self-conscious about singing. His sense of position and his sense of touch are the most acute at this stage, and gently stroking his forehead can be very soothing, too. Harlow's experiment on monkeys with substitute mothers showed that a soft, warm vibrating cloth mother meant more to the little monkey than a wire frame with his food available as he wanted it: He went and got the food when necessary, but he came back to the comforting sensation of the soft, pulsating cloth mother.

As the mother feeds, bathes, changes, carries, cuddles, and talks to her baby, she conveys love in a very practical sense. Every mother will say that her baby needs love, but the baby may not recognize what he is getting as love. Expensive clothes and copious kisses are not felt as love while wet diapers, an empty tummy, and an uncomfortable position go unrelieved. But gentle, prompt attention convinces the baby that his needs will be met, and he learns to wait a little longer once he is sure that his mother is reliable and reasonably consistent.

Here is where the routine comes in, and the predictability of the mother's behavior. Dr. Joost Meerloo, a psychiatric consultant to the United Nations studying the urge to rage and violence, has observed that we should look at the societies that are free of criminals in order to learn how best to control the common phenomenon in our Western civilization. "The innate emotional bomb of violence, uncontrolled rage and self-destructive dying usually explodes when parental and societal care fail. The few societies that are happily free of criminals are characterized by stable inner cohesion, by *lack of early frustration,* as well as by the *total warm ritualistic care and protection* given their citizens from the cradle to the grave."

Appropriate Stimulation

Meerloo also considers that a serious obstruction to normal growth into maturity is related to "too early propulsion into the world" and that the extreme vulnerability of the infant that makes him so dependent on those who care for him can result in resentment and violence if not carefully handled to give the child scope to develop: "Not only do we often hate the hand that feeds us, but we sometimes bite it." Parents must tread a delicate path between overprotection (preventing the child from receiving adequate stimulation and outlet for his energy) and excessive exposure to stimulation that he is not mature enough to handle.

In our Western society it is disturbing to see competitive behavior that leads parents to push a great variety of sieved foods into infants within a few weeks of birth, on the extraordinary assumption that all one needs to consume them is teeth and that, if you have no teeth, then homogenizing achieves the same end—ignoring the lack of readiness of the gastrointestinal tract. I gaze in amazement at the clothes some mothers put on their children—brassiere-topped bikinis on four-year-olds, G-strings on babies who are left exposed in the open sunlight until they have a first-degree burn all over and even a few patches of second degree. There are frightened women who put their daughters on the pill at the onset of menstruation (one even asked me if I thought it would be a good idea to put a crushed pill in her daughter's food daily as she did not wish her to risk pregnancy but did not want to tell her she was on the pill). We see women pushing their children into dating at thirteen and earlier. I heard of a woman recently who saw the principal about her teen-age daughter because she was worried that the girl, though studying and doing well at school, was not interested in having a steady boyfriend. The mother, a divorced socialite, was not worried at all about her other daughter, who was not doing well at school and was quite promiscuous. As I talk to teen-agers, I am very distressed to find how afraid they are of homosexuality. All the publicity given to this minority group has made teen-agers think that any teen-ager seen arm in arm with another of the same sex is homosexual: The cry of "lesbian" follows them around the playground. The congratulatory hug for success at sports or exams is now frowned on by boys and girls, and they have no physical way of demonstrating their friendship and approval. I am sure that this is one of the factors pushing children into earlier sexual experiment. If one is robbed of the normal behavior of the homosexual phase of development one may be almost pushed into too early heterosexual experience.

It is very early in child care that the parents must decide to provide *care suitable for the child's stage of development;* and this "ritualistic" care has to maintain its reliability and regularity but have the flexibility to change to suit developmental needs. It is only too easy to leave the "good" baby in his crib all day and never talk to him; it is also easy to prop a restless baby in front of a TV set and leave him fascinated by flashing lights and strange sounds when the stimulation he should be receiving is his mother's voice and touch.

What kind of child does a TV set rear? I often look at a program and imagine I am a four-year-old or an eight-year-old learning how adults behave. Do try it. You may find that if an adult wants something he takes it, and if resisted he is likely to knock the other man down or hit him in the face. If a man sees an attractive girl he whistles, ogles, and paws, and gets into bed with her as fast as the program can manage it, the girl apparently being flattered and ready to strip at the first invitation. If you are parents who do not act in this way, your child may well decide that it is you who are out of step with the modern world. Ask for the programs you want, protest at programs that are at unsuitable viewing times, and thank the stations that put on good programs.

Common Sense and Experts

One would imagine that food, hygiene, and sleep would follow commonsense lines, common sense being that pool of communal knowledge that indicates predictable results from certain behavior. But far from it! The so-called experts often do not have this ability to recognize common sense, and they may go contrary to nature's most predictable patterns. Perhaps logic is not taught any more. Medical students are exposed to a lot of ivory-tower experts, many of whom would not be able to exist in the outside world. I know no medical course that adequately covers simple nutrition, preparation of food, logical reasoning, normal child development, and normal human sexuality; so one may well find doctors just as kinky on sex and food as the general public.

I think you must know your doctor and not assume that all doctors are equally well trained or reliably informed. This is also the era of individual responsibility. In populations that can read and write, the multitude of popular magazines will supply all the contradictory information you require to choose your own expert, and your child can suffer in the process. If you are a mother who craves precise instructions and follows them slavishly from week to week, then do be sure your authority is well informed. I do not really recommend this method. It is better to learn as much as you can by yourself and have a pediatrician or a general practitioner with special training in pediatrics whose philosophy of life is much the same as yours.

Discussion Groups

It is also a good idea to keep in touch with the other women who went to prenatal classes with you and to form a mothers' discussion group under the leadership of someone well informed in child care. May I warn you here again to avoid the professional group leader who, having often taken a course in the techniques of manipulating people in a group, thinks that he can lead a group in any subject. This can result in some extraordinary pooled ignorance.

To learn and exchange knowledge you need reliable authorities, a good library, and a leader who knows the subject. Such bodies as the La Leche Breast-feeding Council and maternity hospital classes bring together women wanting reliable information on child care and development, and their group leaders are likely to be well informed on the subject as well as on techniques of leading a group. You will appreciate emotional support and encouragement and sharing the experience of learning about children, but I do recommend a child development class rather than a child psychology class: This is not the time to study your child in parts.

In our society, with its small families and isolated units, a woman does not get the knowledge that used to be passed on from generation to generation or the experience of caring for brothers and sisters as she grows up, and she often must get her experience at the same time as she learns the theory. There is a great need for government support of health education programs. For individuals, cash handouts and baby-sitting services are not what is needed to improve child care, and I cannot understand the blindness of government health departments that pour money into family planning, mental health, drug education, abortion clinics, child-care centers, and unsupervised allowances to unmarried teen-agers, but will not support health education programs in maternity hospitals.

Every woman must ask herself: Am I learning enough of the art and science of child care? Am I getting good enjoyable communication with my children and my husband? Am I understanding my children's signals? It is the quality not the quantity of mother's care that counts.

Father

What of father and the first weeks at home? He, too, wants to feel needed and to have contact with his wife and child. He wants to feel that he is protecting them and providing for them, and he can feel very disturbed and left out if he does not have the opportunity to accept this responsibility. If his wife does not need him at this time, she may soon find that someone else has found that she needs him and convinced him that he needs her.

This is a period of adjustment that our society does not recognize as important. Every primitive society has rules and regulations applying to this time in life, but in our society we have employers breaking up families and ignoring their need to be together at crisis times. I have even known large companies to send husbands overseas just as a baby was due, when a little consideration and understanding would have given them a grateful employee instead of a resentful man who would soon be looking for another job. Even the army is more considerate, and the Commonwealth public servants in Australia now get a week's paternity leave.

A man as he looks at his baby feels the same tenderness and purity of affection that his wife feels, and he will cradle the baby just as gently in his arms. The tradition of stiff upper lip has put a false emphasis on hiding emotion as part of masculinity. This generation is much more aware than their parents were of the need to show affection, but often unfortunately less aware of the responsibilities that love requires.

Becoming a father is as important to the man as becoming a mother is to the woman, and father's role in the family is just as important as mother's, not for infant survival but for sexual and social development. It is just as well to get the father involved in baby care right from the beginning. I don't mean that he must get up at night—after all he has to go to work in the morning—but why shouldn't he bathe the baby occasionally and change a diaper?

You have both been through a very great emotional experience and will undoubtedly wish to express your sexual love for each other, and this may need a little finesse and consideration. Tenderness and gentleness are just as important masculine characteristics as courage and strength.

This is a very important time for the marriage, and many marriages begin to fail when the mother comes home with her first baby. She is nervous and emotional; she tires easily and is apt to be weepy and irritable. I remember a young mother saying, "The radiant motherhood business is a myth; I have never been so tired and unhappy in my life." Intercourse my be painful and the new mother anything but satisfactory as a lover; besides, you may wake the baby! That baby comes irritatingly between you, and many men feel an unreasonable jealousy. Father is often tempted to drown his trouble in the usual masculine fashion, in drinking with his friends, and this is not appreciated by his wife. For those whose attitude toward sexual relations has been rather casual and not exclusive before marriage, and who have not learned to discipline their emotions or learned the satisfaction of a continuing exclusive relationship with one person, this really is a dangerous time, and the good-time girl in the office may assume a threatening attractiveness. But this is also a time when a man can really consolidate his marriage and make it so secure that his wife will be eternally grateful and adore him for the rest of her life. Of course, it may mean that father has to take an active interest in the laundry and the shopping. Actually, he finds some shortcuts to getting the work done and does some rearranging of the house to reduce work. It is a very good time for some masterful leadership.

Setting Limits and Guidelines

Everyone who rears a child wants to bring him up to be able to cope with the world, to be happy at least much of the time, to be able to get satisfaction from developing his talents, to be able to form satisfying relationships with other people in friendship and love, and to find an enduring sexual love. We tend to think of what we want for the child rather than of what he will contribute to his world, but that is perhaps the main role of parents: to protect, encourage, and educate, and to help the child find his limitation and his potential. One of the least understood aspects of parental love is that it involves the setting of limits and providing of guidelines at each stage of development. James Baldwin makes this frightening statement: ". . . the child who is not told where the limits are knows, though he may not know that he knows it, that no one cares enough about him to prepare him for his journey."

How to set the necessary limits is the burning question. In conducting a series of discussions with teachers becoming involved in a human relationships program in schools, I gave the first introductory talk on adolescent development, and after we had chatted about various aspects of adolescent behavior I asked the teachers to decide what subjects we would have for our first real discussion. With one voice they chose "discipline."

Of all the subjects parents ask me to speak about, discipline must also be the most common, and as I talk to adolescents their main complaint about parents is, "They are too strict," "They don't understand our need for freedom!" Yet they want the limits set, and they must challenge their parents until they find just where the limits are set if they are to learn the parents' standards and values. I remember an occasion when the daughter of a friend of mine once informed her mother that she and her friends were going to have a night at The Cross (not a religious gathering, but Sydney's center of night life and haunt of all the sex deviants, dropouts, way-outs, and excitement-seekers) and that for this outing she must have the family car. My normally very tolerant friend agonized about it for some time and finally said, "No you are not having the car!" To her amazement her daughter said, "Thank goodness. Now we can't go, and I didn't want to."

To be able to set limits one must understand child development. The very first lesson may be when the baby bites his mother's breast in play and has to choose between getting his meal or misbehaving and hurting his mother. I am sure that all my main mistakes have been due to knowing too much about what can go wrong and not enough about the range of normal behavior and the need for a loose rein. Being a pediatrician is not really the best preparation for parenthood, because one lives in the shadow of fear, having seen what can happen through lack of foresight and guidance; but being a pediatrician makes one aware beyond all doubt that what matters most to a child is a family that cares about him.

So love needs discipline and guidance, but more than that it must be reasonably consistent. How can a child learn how to cope with the world if he lives in an environment that is unpredictable? He will only learn who he is and what he can do and where he is going if the early years teach him what to expect and how to cope with both success and failure, how to pick himself up and laugh and try again. Laughter is a wonderful relaxation from life's tensions, and perhaps one of the great problems of the postwar generations has been their inability to laugh at themselves and the lack of really funny entertainment. They take sex so desperately seriously, with such emphasis on techniques and orgasms, that they are unable to have a good laugh together when the great experience, as it sometimes does, becomes a very funny one. Teen-agers so often turn to violence and horror and drugs as they look for their magical unreality, when it is there for the taking in laughter, love, and fulfillment of potential.

How do you prepare a child for life and teach him how to meet its hazards, particularly when you are very aware of the mistakes you have made and the opportunities you missed? Perhaps they were not always mistakes, perhaps the opportunities were better missed, perhaps it was just life. But, whatever it was, your child is learning how to cope with life as he grows up in the family you provide for him; he is learning your idea of love and the way you show it and he is learning what you laugh at and, above all, he is learning what you value most, or at least the priorities: money, excitement, power, escape from reality, friendship, sex, the family, career, impressing others, or possessions.

Preparing a child for life all comes back to understanding one's own needs and one's own anxieties and ambitions, and to understanding the needs of children at different stages of development, so that parents and children can give one another the support we all need and truly have a liberated family as the basic unit of our society. A family that has true freedom recognizes the rights and needs of others and sets limits; it has patience and love, and takes time to experiment, to gain knowledge, and to use it to improve the quality of life for all.

If the family fails, all the other groups and institutions that care for the child and educate him—school, scouts, sports groups—all have their task made more difficult. Building a sound family is basic to the child's future happiness.

The mother and father have many decisions to make and talk over together. What school is he to attend? What community activity will he take part in? What parent groups will you join? What family leisure activities are possible? Remember Parent Power: It is your only way of influencing education departments and the mass media and even governments. Every parent has a vote, a pen, and a voice. Use them!

10

The Working
Mother

It is strange to realize that everyone reading that heading accepted without question that it referred to women who are members of the work force; yet there is no more time-consuming, tiring job than caring for a home and family. That, indeed, is work. However, this chapter is about work for remuneration.

An increasing number of women are now members of the work force. The Women's Bureau, United States Department of Labor, 1972, gave some rather staggering figures. Working mothers increased from 1.6 million in 1940 to 12.2 million in 1971. "Nearly 7.8 million of these working mothers had children 6 to 17 years of age, 2 million had children 3 to 5 years of age, and 2.3 million had children under 3 years of age. These mothers had a total of 25.7 million children of whom 5.6 million were under 6." In Britain nearly 6 million married women are in the work force. This sounds like a serious situation, involving a great deal of family breakdown and maternal deprivation and possible harm to the children, but we must try to look at it dispassionately.

The working mother receives a lot of criticism and blame. Does she deserve it? If, in the words of the old song, 50 million Frenchmen can't be wrong, can we really say that 12 million American women and 6 million British women must be wrong? Why all the fuss, anyway? In rural communities women help in the fields.

When women are gainfully employed in their own homes at arts and crafts, or when they are out playing golf, do they take better care of their children than if they work in industry? Are social and economic pressures forcing women into situations where they are causing long-term harm to their children without being aware of the risks?

In the last twenty years there have been many reports and conferences on the working mother and her needs and the effect of her work on her children. The Medical Women's International Association has held two international conferences—on the working mother in 1956 and on women in industry in 1970. The World Health Organization has published a report on *Care of Children in Day Care Centers* and also a *Reassessment of the Effects of Deprivation of Maternal Care* (1962). Women's lib has put enormous stress on the right of women to work and be paid.

It is apparent that industrialization and the resultant urbanization of communities break up the wider family pattern. Crowded together in cities, yet in isolated nuclear family units, women have less help with their children than they used to have, yet at the same time, in a cash economy, they need to go out of their homes to obtain paid work. Almost gone is the seamstress doing piecework in her home in her own time. She now must work fixed hours away from her children; she also finds that in buying the products of the factory and the professional she can get more with the cash she earns at her own occupation than if she stayed at home, made the children's clothes, cooked jam, and shelled peas.

Once my own children had reached college age I felt justified in leaving them occasionally to attend international conferences without too great a sense of guilt, provided of course it was not examination time and they were well. These conferences made it very clear to me that the changing role of women has created a worldwide problem. The women of the Third World are now facing the same problem that we have been debating in the West for two decades, but for them the impact is even more sudden. Many of the upper-class Indian and other Asian women, who have always had servants to care for their homes and children, have stepped into professions with apparently few problems. I remember a Filipino professor at a mental health conference getting up and asking in amazement what was all the fuss about leaving children at home: Her children were with her family and servants and there was no worry. Hearing the Africans express great concern at the effect of the transistor radio promoting Western goods and culture in every village, and at the deterioration of nutrition in infants as women abandoned breast-feeding to go to work, made one aware of a deep disquiet at the change occurring in family patterns in the developing countries.

It has been both exciting and frightening to listen to doctors in communist countries and Israel, where the building of new societies has received first priority and where the task of caring for the children of women required in the work force has been tackled methodically and child-care facilities have been provided—exciting, because these countries faced the need for adequate substitute care and aimed at and achieved an improvement in material and educational standards for a majority of children; frightening, because this is how children can be indoctrinated and prepared for a new way of life and regimes that are difficult to change. Wars and mass movements of population separated children from parents and gave them varying types of substitute care at different ages; the experts have now had opportunities to study the results—the writings of Spitz, Bowlby, Roudinesco, Anna Freud, Robinson, Ainsworth, Bettelheim, the fascinating discussion on *Determinants of Infant Behaviour*, and many other publications are now available.

Many conflicting conclusions emerge that often fail to differentiate between the effect of urban living, of broken homes, of separation from the mother at an early age, and of whether the mother was working or not; but it is quite apparent that there are dangers and advantages for both mothers and children in mothers taking employment outside their homes. "The emotional problems of children may be found repeatedly to be related, not to the mother's employment status but to her own emotional state." It may well be worse for a child to spend twenty-four hours a day in the care of an unloving woman, inexperienced in child care, or of an obsessive housekeeper, or in an atmosphere of smother love, than even eight hours a day in a well-run day-care center with a responsible and responsive staff.

The International Labour Office reports: "Experience in a

number of countries suggests that many mothers of young children prefer to stay at home while their children are small if they are in a position to do so and the prevailing opinion is that the presence of the mother is particularly important where there are young children unless alternative arrangements assure them the type of care and affection they need." It is quite clear that the younger the child, the more vulnerable he is, and that it is the quality rather than the quantity of mothering the child receives that matters. The New South Wales Branch of the Australian and New Zealand College of Psychiatrists prepared a memorandum on some aspects of the welfare of children under three years old whose mothers are in full-time employment. They strongly advised against full-time work for the mothers of these children. Not only is there difficulty in finding good substitute care, but "it does not give the mother a chance to develop her own relationship with her young child."

The family woman, busy at home with her household and normally not politically inclined, is now rising in wrath and demanding why women who either choose or have been forced to hand over their family responsibilities to others should be rewarded when the family woman gets less help and no pay and her husband pays taxes.

Let us look at why women are going back to the work force in such large numbers and see if some constructive suggestions can be made to find a compromise between conflicting interests.

International conference reports and national statistics show that women with husbands are much less likely to reenter the work force while their children are young or to take on full-time employment; so the overwhelming answer to why women work is an economic and not an ideological one. For the vast majority of women home, husband, and children come first, and it is primarily in their material interests that a woman goes out to earn money rather than because she needs adult company or is ambitious in her profession

Shortage of money is not a problem just of the lower-income groups. What many people fail to realize is that the professional and middle-income groups find that marriage, with two living on the wage of one, makes a very sudden change in their way of life. Though the income can still appear adequate, the couple has moved into a very different income bracket, and to maintain their standard of living, particularly if they are buying a home, the woman must go to work. The fact that the income would be adequate for many people makes no difference to how they feel about it.

Another financial reason is often that, no matter how cooperative her husband may be about the housekeeping money, clothing allowances, etc., it is not easy for a woman who has been earning her own money to accept a weekly allowance from him. Somehow it does affect the relationship, and most women want to have some money of their own to use as they like, regardless of how well the partnership works. Don't imagine that they want to spend it on themselves: I know women with accounts for children's education, family vacations, and other family activities. It does a great deal for a woman's morale to have her own money, even if she pays it into a joint account.

In a materialistic society such as Western civilization of the New World type, a money value is placed on everything, and even the most dedicated, idealistic mother is unable to suppress her envy as her smartly dressed neighbor leaves in her own car to take her child to the day nursery on her way to work; she often bitterly attacks her neighbor's way of life. When working time is valued at so many dollars an hour, the mother who is not receiving payment in cash for her services to her family not only experiences the financial pinch but feels herself to be of less value than the paid employee. Women educated in the same way as men and trained in highly skilled occupations feel this even more; they have a contribution to make to society, they have skills to be used, and they need to use them to see themselves as worthwhile people.

Another important factor in women working outside their homes is the nature of Western society. Suburbia, with its individual houses and competitive "keep up with the Joneses" type of home furnishing, is unfriendly and lonely and a big contrast to our peer-group type of educational system. From the age of three and a half to sixteen, or even to twenty-five for some college students, our children are thrown into the peer group; it is almost an educator's obsession to keep children in their own age group. So after fifteen years of this type of suppression of individuality, of set syllabuses and of academic education, with little education in human relationships and the arts and crafts of everyday living, the isolation of being at home all day with a child is a great contrast. The housewife feels trapped—loving her husband, desperately anxious to give her child the best she can, but seeing herself as a different person from the woman who earned a living and was independent. She sees that changed woman being irritable, resentful, and hurtful to the family she loves, shouting at them and appearing an ugly person. She also finds that with the household aids of a technological age, such as washing machines, dishwashers, a hot-water supply, vacuum cleaners, stainless-steel sinks, and steam irons, she can maintain a high standard of home care in a much shorter time than her mother did. She has a smaller family, and her pregnancies are planned. The supermarket, one-stop shopping with all the miracles of canned, prepackaged, and frozen foods, ready-made clothing, and even home delivery can be a great boon to her. It is unfortunate that our educational system and industry do not cooperate better to prepare her and her husband for home management in the technological age, because their lack of knowledge of nutrition, budgeting, and human relationships can result in a lower standard of family care.

Some women who feel inadequate for the task of caring for a family, and compare this inadequacy with their former efficiency in employment, are now thinking that they are failures and are being brainwashed into going back to work by the argument that it is better to leave the job of child and family care to the experts than to demand education to help them do a more satisfying job themselves. These women are being made to feel resentful and inferior by the noisy extremists of the women's liberation movement who are trying to escape from child care, family responsibility—and their own womanhood. Self-centered, unloving, and often insecure women who have failed in human relationships may still be very good at their jobs in the work force and are apt to be militant liberationists. I have met brilliant academics and business women and factory workers who reject the traditional female role, putting their own "freedom" before the welfare of their husbands and children. Often such women have had an unhappy childhood without parental concern, and personal experience of abortion and broken marriage; so they want to destroy what others have found a successful and joyful way of life in the full acceptance of what mature womanhood can mean. A movement that downgrades homemaking skills, abandons children to state care, and blames men for all female trouble is not going to raise the status of women.

The Single-Parent Family

Some special consideration must be given to the single-parent family. Whether that parent is male or female, there are many problems. Let us here consider the woman who is trying to rear her children without their father's day-to-day assistance. She must inevitably obtain regular paid employment if she is even to approach the standard of living that could have been expected with her husband, and she has a more difficult task in every way than the woman with an interested husband. Not only has she the full responsibility of the children with their daily demands and distresses, but she must cope with the minor catastrophes that fathers usually attend to—like leaking taps, flat tires, and blown fuses, and the major problems of income tax and the garden. Frequently she is getting little alimony, or fears to press for it because of the added emotional stress if the children are regularly accessible to what she believes is undesirable paternal influence. She has a constant fear of illness and the loss of her job, and of what may be happening to her children when her job has to take first priority.

Many personal problems face the deserted wife, the widow, and the divorcee who sincerely entered marriage as a lifelong commitment "till death do us part" and found that she had made an impossible contract, or that her partner had merely pledged "until another do us part." Not only are her own emotional needs inadequately met, but society regards her with suspicion, particularly if she is attractive and dresses well. With other women casting a wary eye in her direction and clutching their husbands to them, she often finds her social life very restricted: cut off from the kind of mixed male and female company of her former life, dropped from guest lists, and regarded as fair game by the office Don Juan. She can be very lonely.

The number of single-parent families is increasing and more research is needed into why this is happening. Women say they prefer to cope alone rather than expose themselves and their children to alcoholic, violent, or unfaithful husbands, and I am sure there will be more men refusing to tolerate unfaithful and unsatisfactory wives when the women's liberationists get their way and achieve the kind of equality in marriage that removes protection of women. When a man can show that he cares for his children and can provide just as good a day-care center as the working mother, there seems no reason why she should get custody of the children as easily as she has in the past.

No New Phenomenon

The woman working to contribute to the support of her home and family has always been the norm throughout the ages. It is no new phenomenon, at least in Judeo-Christian culture. In Proverbs we read of the good wife: She worked at home weaving the children's clothing and bed covers, she worked in her garden, she sold the goods she did not need, she was a good business woman. "After careful thought, she buys a field and plants a vineyard out of her earnings." A real working mother! But she met the needs of her husband and children too: "her husband's whole trust is in her" and "her sons with one accord call her happy." "Like a ship laden with merchandise she brings food from afar off" . . . not modern woman coming home from the supermarket but the woman of ancient Israel! We sound like a feeble lot beside her, or do we?

What is a new phenomenon is the woman isolated in her home, unable to make a financial or equivalent contribution to the material welfare of her family unit, not educated to do it, and with government, industry, and women who envy men trying to devalue what she can do and force her out to work. The other new phenomenon is the nature of the new society that has reduced the value of the household arts by making the products readily available in the supermarket and inundating women with glossy magazines that set impossible standards for household furnishing and cooking, rather than stressing basic needs. We want to have the satisfaction of the woman of ancient Israel and her family restored, but fulfilled in a modern way: That is what I call Family Liberation.

From work in the community women can gain financially and

raise the standard of living; they can also gain socially and emotionally. It is shown that they suffer less from the "empty-nest syndrome" of depression when the families grow up and leave home. I am sure also that they are less interfering mothers-in-law and more understanding of modern youth. The mother of two needs an active interest, whether remunerative or not. The real question is not whether she should go back to work but what the outside interest should be, when she should take it up, and what the dangers are to herself and to her family.

It is not always morale building to go back to work. Too often the mother finds that the market considers her unreliable, likely to take time off whenever her children need her, wanting to work hours that suit her family; she is offered inferior positions and less pay than men and is passed over for men with inferior qualifications. According to statistics, absenteeism is not greater among working mothers and they take fewer sick days. These women are usually more responsible. They have home responsibilities and the job is important to them, so they work hard, and they don't pretend to be sick or go slow, because they want the job near home and jobs are not easy for them to get. It is, however, a fact that most women who have families do not seek employment of a very responsible nature until their children are at school. Some interesting studies of women in industry have shown that mothers of young children often do routine work that is quite boring and repetitive, even though they are capable of doing much more responsible work. This may be because the emotional stresses of caring for a young family do not leave much ambition and initiative available at that time. Every real mother of a young child is never far away from it in her thoughts.

What Are the Dangers to the Woman?

Fatigue as she tackles two jobs is probably the greatest danger for the working mother. It can weaken relationships within the family so that her husband and children can stray to find love elsewhere; she can fail to become a wife and mother emotionally. A man working in this competitive society needs to be able to relax and feel comforted when he comes home. A tired, irritable wife trying to cope at night with the housework that has not been done may soon find her family life in difficulties and herself resentful of the husband who is not helping. She will also feel guilty as she meets the prejudice of the world, both male and female, though this is getting less. Whatever ills befall her, she will wonder if going to work was the cause.

It is also not easy to recognize changes in oneself. Absorbed in more outside activities, you do not realize that the children are not talking to you about school and their problems, and that they are playing away from home.

Doctors and schoolteachers will tend to ascribe all the bad behavior of her offspring to the mother going to work, even if the father is no help. If the child happens to stammer or get asthma or wet the bed, some doctor will assure her that it is all the result of her going to work, in spite of the complete lack of statistical proof that these conditions are even emotional in origin. In fact, there is no statistical evidence that women who are working mothers have more maladjusted children than mothers who stay at home, and there is considerable evidence that the children of working mothers find their mothers more interesting and life more challenging. Evaluating the effect of women being at work is very difficult, since so many of the women supposedly at home are at the club playing cards or on the golf course, or the baby is propped in front of the TV set while the mother does the housework or chats to a neighbor or even entertains a boyfriend.

Most mothers want only part-time work. The mother who has full-time employment as well as a home and family is inevitably very tired, unless she has full-time domestic help. If she has a very cooperative husband who helps with the domestic chores, then all may be well, but most women with children want part-time work that they can do within school hours, and neither unions nor employers are willing to give them such work—though employers are more willing to do so than the unions.

The Dangers to the Child

I am often asked by mothers contemplating going to work what is best for the children. Some quickly rationalize and convince themselves that the washing machine or the new furniture they will buy with the money is much more important than their presence in the home; but I am often involved in helping to plan the best type of child care for the woman who feels she must go back to work and in helping her decide at what age she can expose her child to the risk. What risk? The risk that her child may accept a substitute mother instead of her? The risk that the substitute mother may not be reliable and the child become confused and unable to develop lasting relationships? The risk that separation from mother may have quite far-reaching emotional effects that cause recurrent problems? The risk of repeated respiratory-tract infections, ear, nose, and throat infections, viruses passed around the day nursery? They are all very real risks for the child under three.

THE QUALITY OF CHILD CARE

The greatest problem in providing child-care facilities is to obtain the right kind of staff. "Gentleness, patience and above all love of children are essential and no technical competence can make up for the absence of these qualities" (WHO report); but technical training is very important. For the baby and infant a high standard of hygiene and first aid, a good appreciation of illness and health, and a good knowledge of child development and behavior are essential. The staff will be handling many children; it is easy for infection to spread. Infants need love, security, close physical contact, and the opportunity to attach to one person; they need routine. The two-to-five-year-old needs a lot of stimulation; he is aware of color, texture, variations in sound; he is learning control of his body, balancing, riding bikes and rocking horses; he is copying those around him and learning how to respond to people and provoke responses from them. From the staff in a day-care center that the child attends all day he will learn language, reaction patterns, and habits of hygiene; he will develop a close relationship with them and model himself on them; and he will learn attitudes that will affect his later learning. It is certainly not enough to have a kindly soul who had reared her own ten children in charge of children in a child-care center; she must have professional training, maybe a simple short course for assistants, but a full child-care course for the women in charge.

I believe in the importance of establishing child-care facilities for the children of all mothers, not only part-time and full-time working mothers but the harassed housewife who badly needs some outside interest or cannot face the battle of the supermarket when junior disappears around the showcases and pulls the bottom can from the towering display of soup with crashing results. If it is to be government policy to provide child-care facilities, and it seems that it is essential to do so, then the first priority is well-trained staff that will be alert to the child's needs and be able to guide the mother in how to meet them. Let me make a few dogmatic but generally accepted statements on these needs.

THE IMPORTANCE OF THE FIRST THREE YEARS

The first three years of life are critical for the formation of a warm, secure mother-child relationship and during that period there is no great need for the company of other children of the same age. The baby is learning fast from his mother and father all the time and often gets accustomed to another baby. Separations at this time may be very disturbing.

The play-group movement, through which mothers meet together and pool play equipment and ideas to provide stimulation and security for their children, is greatly enriching the lives of mothers and children and helping them to independence without separating them from each other.

It is better for a child not to be separated all day from his mother until he can talk and is toilet trained. In fact, if the mother has to go to work before this time she should make every effort to be with her child for as many meals as possible, for his bath, and to settle him down to sleep; this obviously means that I think it is better that mothers should not attempt outside work except for short periods with an infant under two years. The management of sleep, feeding, elimination of waste, and general hygiene is so closely associated with the emotional development and responsiveness of a child that the woman who hands this job over to another is handing over her normal role of adapting the environment to his needs and teaching him habits. She is also missing these stages of development, missing opportunities to learn his signals for aid; so she is not developing as a mother herself.

Biographies of some of the well-known British peers reared by

nannies make it quite clear that it was nanny who got their affection and molded their attitudes. A child learns affection,
communication, habits, and a set of values from the woman who
taught him as a baby, plus what is added by teachers. It must be
quite apparent that often the natural parents are not imparting
even their values and habits, and, what is more, they are not
learning to communicate with their children. All animals have
signals that the young must learn if they are to communicate and
survive—smell, touch, sound, facial expression, awareness of
movement. Before a child learns speech, communication is on this
level, too, and a child is more aware of the warmth and nearness
of the person and the tone of the voice than of the words. If the
mother does not learn to communicate at the level of touch and
sound and transfer of emotion I do not think she ever becomes
that child's mother in the full meaning of the word. I am also sure
that most women can learn these signals and learn to respond to
their children. All the signals are related to survival, loving,
eating, sleeping, and elimination, and I do not think it is so very
difficult for a woman who wants to keep up her profession and
technical skill to plan their use in such a way as not to harm her
child.

Much depends on the nature of the woman's training and her
sensitivity to the needs of her husband and child, and if she gets
her priorities right, well-planned periods of separation from her
child can help to develop his independence: "The ability to cope
with the environment on one's own is essential to growth and
development and would seem to depend, in part, on mild doses of
separation and large doses of opportunity to develop one's own
initiative" (Leona Baumgartner, at the Medical Women's International Association 12th Congress, 1970).

INFLUENCING THE YOUNG CHILD

There is great need for men and women of integrity who care
about children and the future of the race; who wish to see all
children given full opportunities in education and work, and a
high standard of values by which to live and learn to love. The
pronouncements of some of the full-time academics and ad-
ministrators who sit in their offices and ivory towers and play

with people's lives are, to me, appalling and dangerous. They appear to assume that all people want the same things. Academic doctors in Communist China at least have to spend a fixed period each year working in the communes to see how people live—which must make them understand people better.

Women with families are much more aware than our academics of the needs of children and of mothers, and Western society will have to find means of meeting the needs of the working mother, both through employers in industry and through government measures. Soviet society, setting up a system by which everyone works for the government, has provided child-care facilities that meet the needs of the mother and child adequately. The Soviet has modified its original ideas on marriage and abortion and child care. While I was in Moscow I had an opportunity to talk to some women and there seemed to be a very real awareness of the value of the family and the needs of children and the acceptance of a high sexual moral code to preserve that family. Modern Israel has set up systems of child care that have enabled women to work for their country. Japan has an industrialized society where the big private corporations have developed a paternalistic system.

Surely we can learn by studying all these—always bearing in mind that as soon as any centralized organization takes over the care of children, the power to mold their lives goes into the hands of a few people; this, of course, is the way to produce a society that is easy to control and dominate.

The younger the child, the greater the effect of standardized care in suppressing the uniqueness of the individual. We do need child-care facilities—emergency, casual, and regular—but all parents must remain deeply involved in the care of their children and know just what is happening to them: What kind of people are molding their children, what kind of training are they being given? Parents need to continue their own education in child care and to have facilities to do so.

Essentials for Working Mothers

I think a few clear statements can be made that would be generally accepted by the child-care authorities.

The highest priority is to establish a warm, trusting, and enjoyable relationship between father, mother, and child, and this must involve father as early as possible in the day-to-day family living. It means, for infants up to three years, that the mother should be the main provider of daily care. In the one-to-three-year period a play group will broaden the experience and pleasure of mother and child, and part-time day care by a well-trained woman can be satisfactory. There is an enormous difference between all-day care and consistent care for a few hours that does not alter the child's day-to-day routine management of feeding, sleeping, and elimination. Preschool for three-to-five-year-olds (i.e., from 9:00 A.M. to 3:30 P.M.) with trained teachers is of advantage to most children; but it is not necessarily the best care, depending on the family. I have seen mothers going to work to pay for preschool services, when they did not want to but thought it essential that the child go to preschool.

If the mother can have part-time work from 9:00 till 3:00 for one or two days a week, then this usually works out very well; but when she starts at 7:00 A.M. or comes home from 5:00 to 7:00 P.M. problems will soon arise. Women who have work they can do at home, or part-time work for a few hours at a time, can plan it to suit themselves and can organize it very well even with a small baby; but three months after the birth should be the earliest for starting any employment.

If you can arrange to be home to feed the baby, bathe it, and put it to bed, then you are making excellent contact, and all you have to remember is to get enough rest yourself and not to neglect your husband.

THE MOTHER SUBSTITUTE

If you must return to work full time with a child under two years, you are choosing a mother substitute for your baby and you cannot expect to be first with the child; but the child need not suffer. The mother substitute must be an affectionate, responsible person and the child must have consistent care; mothers who leave their young children with a series of different people, whoever is available, may be disturbing the child's development emotionally and socially. This is also one of the problems in day-care centers. It is not easy to find one where the staff is allocated to particular children that they get to know, and often there are many staff changes that confuse and upset a child. The child may just be getting attached to one person when he loses her, and after this has occurred a few times the child hesitates to give his love to anyone and certainly it will be difficult for him to find security and trust in adults.

I have known mothers who deliberately leave their child with a variety of baby-sitters, saying that they would not like the child to become fond of anyone else but the mother. This is cruel and dangerous. The only responsible thing for a woman to do is to decide that either she undertakes most of her child's care or she finds a reliable and consistent substitute. Caring for children is highly skilled work; to do it well requires knowledge of child behavior, nutrition, preparation of food, hygiene, first aid, as well as patience and a warm responsive personality. I am constantly amazed at how women expect to get this kind of service cheaply. It staggers me to think that an expert committee on child care could have recommended that a good way to mind children for women going to work is to find motherly, experienced women who can mind six children at a time in their own homes by themselves all day. I wilt at the thought, but I stiffen again in anger at the suggestion that no training is required for such a task!

The best arrangement is probably a day-care center at or near the place of employment, so that the mother can go to the child at lunchtime and possibly at other short breaks. Such a center can be designed to provide all facilities for a number of children more conveniently than a home, and the staff can be allocated to particular children in small groups so that they really get to know the children and the children to know and love them. The younger the children, the more staff needed. Babies need to be fed and changed more frequently, and they should not be left to cry. Some babies are much more restless than others and need more attention; their hygiene and food preparation must be more carefully attended to and they are more helpless. If the baby is not well or has an accident then the risks of serious trouble are greater.

I often find that mothers seem to think having a baby looked after will be cheaper and easier than having a two- or three-year-old looked after. Far from it! It is a more responsible job than most others, and you do not hand your precious baby to someone else to care for while you work without very careful thought and evaluation of the situation.

There are women who find it very hard to give babies good care. Among these are some professional and business women who can afford to pay a nurse and may serve their child better by doing so, and by having short periods of caring for the child they may learn to love. They need not feel guilty about how they feel so long as a suitable nurse is available and they face the reality of the situation. Women who cannot earn a high enough income to employ a nurse may find it much better to arrange with a friend who also has a small child to share a job. This has been tried out in various occupations, such as nursing; it enables both mothers to have a part-time job, and each knows that her child is well cared for by the other while she works. If one child or mother is sick there can be a special arrangement for one mother to work longer. This suits employers, too, but unions have not accepted the idea.

ORGANIZATION AND PLANNING

Any working mother must be well organized, and women repeatedly tell me that going back to work has been very good for them and all the family because they have had to set to and plan the housework, the washing, and the meals, and have found that they can manage it all very efficiently, that they are not nearly so obsessive about tidiness and elaborate meals, and that everyone is happier. They have found that the normal household jobs, like cleaning the bathroom, vacuum-cleaning the carpet, and washing the kitchen floor, can quite satisfactorily be done less often. What really matters is to have a timetable and stick to it. Then you do not suddenly find that the carpet beetles have settled in, and you can look with equanimity at the mess in the kitchen and say, "Well tomorrow is the day for the kitchen," and know that tomorrow all will be well. Living in chaos every day is an impossible situation; it is necessary to see patches of daylight and order and an overall pattern for existence.

ESTABLISHING TRUST

Just a few other important points about children and working mothers. Children of all ages should know where their mother is and where she works. She must never sneak out; she must always say good-bye so that they know she will come back. It is pathetic to see a child searching for mommy, even at fifteen months, just because she did not say good-bye; better to have a good screaming match and be welcomed back, and soon the child realizes that you never go without telling him. It is also better for a parent—and not a friend or neighbor—to leave the child at the day-care center.

Grandparents, of course, are wonderful mother substitutes, but remember that they tire more easily and find it hard to cope for a whole day. They may not be as strong or well as they used to be, but they love their grandchildren and will take better care of them than most other people. One major problem will be that grandmother may not agree with the staff at the day-care center.

PRIORITIES

The mother who is going to work when she has a child under three must examine her priorities very carefully and also her capacity to be a twenty-four-hour-a-day mother. Father may be able to give the child a lot of his time, and fathers can be objects of attachment and provide the warm human relationship that is so necessary to develop warm, responsive human beings. Make sure you can answer these questions:

How important is it that I go to work?

What is my real reason for going back to work?

Have I done everything possible to make it part-time work that fits in with the home routine?

Am I putting the overall welfare of my family first and the needs of my children before my own?

Does my husband agree that I should go to work and is he willing to help at home?

Mothers Who Stay at Home

Somewhat reluctantly I have come to the conclusion that mothers who stay at home to care for their young children should have an allowance from government sources to allow them to stay home if they are in financial need; but I do think that such allowances should be conditional on the child's getting good care, and that means the mother must be subject to some kind of supervision and even attend child-care classes. Perhaps the fairest way to see that the woman who stays at home to care for the house and children is not discriminated against would be to grant tax concessions to the husband. Certainly I think casual child-care facilities should be available to help the normal everyday devoted mother who inevitably does find it tiring to have twenty-four-hour responsibility. Supportive services and facilities and education in child care should have first claim on government finance.

Dr. Margaret Mead says: "We've learned a great deal in the last fifteen years about how human beings are made into human beings by the warmth and closeness of the relationships they have to the people who rear them; but we're going to have to think all this over anew—think it over and reassess what we mean by human warmth, what we mean by ties created between human beings: ties that are based on a permanent sex relationship and the kind of complementary interdependence that we have used as the basis of marriage."

Some mothers make the tie to the child too close; many mothers who go to work too early do not establish a satisfactory tie at all; and an increasing number of women seem to think that the tie with father is not important or that a weekly visit will do. No mother should regard the decision on whether to go to work as one she makes on her own; it may be more important to work on the marriage and develop it into a worthwhile marriage. As Dr. Mead says, we must reassess and rethink our values. The days of following traditional patterns are gone, but the basic values have not changed nor have the basic needs of children.

Education for Mothers

Dr. Whitten, studying underweight children in Detroit, found that the majority were actually receiving insufficient food or unsuitable food. He believed that the term *neglect* was not appropriate, because the mothers did not deliberately neglect their children but "rather they are unaware of their children's needs or their roles in creating the problem or they were unable to respond to their children's needs because they are so preoccupied and consumed by their own conflicts in unsatisfied emotional and situational needs." Money and financial allowances are not the solution for such mothers or families; money spent on health education and advisory services available to all the community is money better spent.

The working mother inevitably feels guilty. She need not so long as she understands her child, puts his needs first, and enjoys him. She often tries to overcome her guilt by spending money on her baby—expensive toys, elaborate clothes, disposable diapers, the best carriage on the street—but these do not make up for lack of loving care by father and mother in an atmosphere of happiness and unity in the family home.

11

Family Planning

Now you are a family—father, mother, and child. You are in business: the business of rearing a child and his future brothers and sisters until they can support themselves. This is a partnership. The man-woman relationship can be the strongest of all ties between two human beings, and now is a good time to give some thought to how soon you want another child, how many you plan to have, and what spacing you wish.

There has been so much emphasis on sex in drama, art, and ballet, on TV, and in the popular magazines that it has become almost axiomatic that if a marriage is not a success from the point of view of sexual satisfaction quite early in its history then it should be dissolved regardless of a child's need for both parents or the ability of two people to restore and develop a relationship that will eventually become a very satisfying one. The obsession with orgasm has greatly disturbed many women who were perfectly happy loving their husbands and not experiencing any world-shattering sensation; and it has made some husbands feel they were failures because they were unable to arouse this sensation.

More research and more detailed records from normal people are making it quite clear that there is a wide variety of responsiveness and of satisfaction, that the most satisfying sexual relationship is a progressive relationship with one person. It interested me to read the review of a book called *Original Skin* by Hansen that surveyed the "social, cultural and countercultural strands that led to the permissiveness of 1970 in art, films, and other art forms," and commented on different experimental forms and sensational presentations of sex. The writer made this observation at the end: "True eroticism is the monopoly of the monogamous couple, enabling them to live together without loss of love or desire. The nonpersonal sex that is being hawked and will continue to be hawked in even greater quantities is a substitute and escape from life, not a means of transcending it."

Real sexual enjoyment of each other is not what the books tell you or what the blue movie implies or attempts to show; it is the exquisite appreciation of each other as individuals, the awareness of each other's presence, the delight of touch and exploring and responsiveness as you learn each other's needs and sources of pleasure. This must inevitably be a progressive and developing relationship that involves total personality. To separate sex from the whole relationship makes it superficial and even impersonal. Desire will fluctuate, and business worries, fatigue, and anxiety about the baby will affect this sensitive area of human relationship, so that any imagined or real rejection or lack of response may become a major cause of friction without even being discussed. So intense and so important is this relationship that husbands and wives often fail to talk about their pleasure and their love and their need for each other, and hurt each other instead. Just as the child who is jealous of the new baby becomes naughty and destructive to make sure he is noticed, so adults can behave in a similar childish fashion without being aware of their problem.

Yes, this is a don't-let-this-happen-to-you introduction to birth control. Too many marriages break up these days because of the false image being presented by the media and by psychologists, because of the modern passion for instant everything, even instant sexual perfection. Those who have this "true eroticism" do not talk about it to others; it is a personal secret—too personal to talk about—and rarely stressed in the marriage manuals so obsessed with techniques.

Recently I read an article by Professor Maslow, a sociologist who had the delightful idea of studying happy people to find out

190 Birth of a Family

what they had in common. Tolstoy once said that all happy families were happy in the same way, and the unhappy ones had an infinite number of ways of being unhappy; but I had never before seen an analysis of the characteristics that were shared by happy people. Well, here are Professor Maslow's observations, and he called his happy people "self-actualizers." They were people who were able to be themselves and achieve realistically, and they shared these characteristics:

1. Commitment to work: What they did they did with enthusiasm and commitment—no tentative tries or "trial marriages" for them; commitment and determination to make a success of the undertaking.
2. Self-acceptance: No pining for what might have been; they accepted their own limitations, they grew old gracefully, they did not pretend success when it was not there; and they enjoyed their emotions and accepted their feelings.
3. They could tolerate uncertainty and venture into the unknown.
4. They were realistic: They recognized the fake and dishonest and the fraud; they loved the genuine article and they faced reality.
5. They had a capacity for appreciation: They appreciated people, beauty, and the world around them; they could be "surprised by joy"; they could sink into the wonder of the universe and be one with it.

Such people can give of themselves and they have a sense of values that goes far beyond self-interest; and these are all attitudes that can be learned and practiced.

What has all that to do with developing this sexual bond that is to last a lifetime and be the greatest relationship one has with another human? A lot! Because Professor Maslow expresses better than I do just what that relationship has to include, and I too would put commitment first.

So often one hears people saying they are not getting what they want out of their marriage. The obvious response is to ask what they are putting into it, and with what sense of commitment to it.

But what of the practical details? If it is decided that this is an exclusive relationship, then it means some synchronizing of sexual desire, something that is not always easy, and the problem is likely to arise sooner after you come home from the hospital than the doctor said it would. The way most obstetricians so cheerfully say, "No intercourse for six weeks before the baby is due, nor for six weeks after," shows a quite incredible lack of understanding of the emotions of the monogamous couple who love each other and have just gone through a truly earth-shattering experience. Even if the husband has been separated from his wife for only a few days in actual time, the separation has been much greater in some other dimension: There is a child between them now, and there is a great need to restore their oneness and to express with their bodies what they often cannot express in words. But episiotomies are painful, and this pseudomodern obstetrics has certainly delayed resumption of intercourse. I hope the fashion soon goes. However, there is still petting to orgasm, and intercourse can be gentle and hygienic and still satisfying.

In the first weeks, if the mother is breast-feeding, there should be no risk of pregnancy, but perhaps to make quite sure it is wise to decide on the method of birth control very soon, and a condom with lubricant for the vagina is probably best. At this early stage there is only one pill that does not have some effect on lactation, and it is less reliable than the others and not as readily available. Most obstetricians do not recommend the use of hormone pills again until ten weeks after delivery. This is a time of hormonal stabilization and returning to normal, and it would seem quite irrational to add a hormonal pill to complicate adjustment. Perhaps this is the time to look at birth control generally, so that you can think more clearly about what you will use.

Birth Control

The main factors to be considered are how you feel about the methods described; whether you have a philosophical or religious objection to some; the convenience; the cost; the side effects; the extent to which you are prepared to take precautions and to practice self-control and avoid ovulation time; and, most important, who is to take the precautions—the man or the woman, or both. Undoubtedly you have already considered the question of birth control in the short term, but now you have to consider the twenty or more years ahead and how you will meet each other's sexual needs without having more children than you can offer a satisfactory life to.

We can consider the methods available under several headings:

1. Avoidance of intercourse during the fertile time of the woman's menstrual cycle.
2. Prevention of ovum and sperm from coming in contact by methods which destroy the sperm and/or prevent its entrance into the uterus.
3. Rendering the male or female infertile by suppressing ovulation or spermatogenesis or, permanently, by sterilization.
4. Preventing implantation of the fertilized ovum.

There are also many who maintain that abortion by deliberate destruction of the implanted ovum or the developing embryo should be legally available as a method of birth control to all who find they have an inconvenient pregnancy.

Physiology of Reproduction

To understand just how these methods work one must first understand the menstrual cycle and what controls it. The menstrual cycle or reproductive cycle is controlled chemically by a beautiful balance between the hypothalamus, pituitary gland, and ovaries, and is regulated by the hormone levels in the blood maintained by interaction of these glands. The cycle starts at the first day of menstruation and in most women is twenty-eight days, sometimes longer, sometimes shorter. It is mostly regular, but variations can occur as a result of emotion, climate, health, and stimulation from higher brain centers. The cycle begins when the hypothalamus releases hormones known as gonadotrophic-releasing hormones that stimulate the pituitary to pour gonadotrophic hormones into the bloodstream. One of these (follicle-stimulating hormone, FSH) acts on the ovary, stimulating egg follicles to grow and start to mature and the ovary itself to produce estrogen, one of the female sex hormones. Estrogen is carried to the uterus by the bloodstream and there it stimulates the lining of the uterus (endometrium) to thicken and get ready to receive the ovum for implantation if it is fertilized after ovulation. Usually only one follicle matures fully, but some women have a

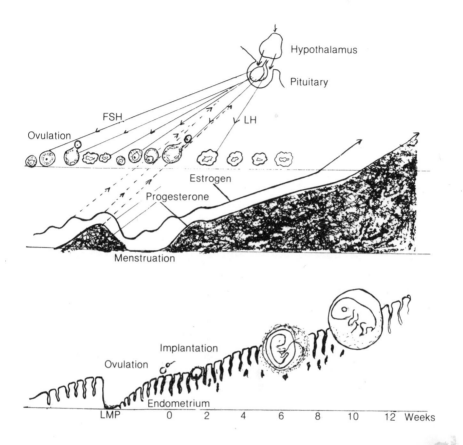

Hypothalamus

Pituitary

FSH

LH

Ovulation

Estrogen

Progesterone

Menstruation

Implantation

Ovulation

Endometrium

LMP   0   2   4   6   8   10   12   Weeks

HORMONES AND THE MENSTRUAL CYCLE

The diagram represents maturation of a follicle, ovulation and development of the corpus luteum for one menstrual cycle, with fertilization and implantation occurring in the next month. Blood levels of estrogen (formed by ovary and placenta) and progesterone (formed by corpus luteum of the ovary, adrenal gland, and placenta) are shown. They have a feedback effect on the pituitary gland to control the menstrual cycle. The effect of the contraceptive pill is to confuse feedback and prevent ovulation. The pituitary secretes follicle-stimulating hormone and luteinizing hormone to stimulate estrogen and progesterone formation. The hypothalamus secretes releasing hormones.

tendency, usually familial, to bring more than one to maturity; and this can lead to two ova being fertilized at once to produce nonidentical twins that can be of different sexes. Identical twins occur when one egg divides, and they are of the same sex. As the estrogen level rises in the blood it causes feedback stimulation of the hypothalamus, and by about fourteen days the pituitary has passed out enough of the second gonadotrophic hormone (luteinizing hormone, LH) into the blood to cause the ovarian follicle to rupture and release its egg. This is quickly caught by waving tentacles on the end of the Fallopian tube and passed along it.

By now the lining of the uterine wall has thickened and the glands of the neck of the uterus (cervix) are producing clear mucus, which will help carry the sperm and keep it moist so it can survive longer. The luteinizing hormone stimulates the ruptured follicle to become a corpus luteum, which produces the second female sex hormone, progesterone. Now the progesterone level in the blood rises. It stimulates the mucous glands to make the mucus thick and cloudy and less copious, and it also affects the breasts and glands in the skin and vagina, and alters body metabolism so that there is a tendency to retain fluid in the tissues. Many women in the postovulation time find that they put on weight, that the breasts and nipples are sensitive, and that they are emotionally less stable; some may experience premenstrual tension. By now the endometrium is thick and ready for implantation; the luteinizing hormone and progesterone levels in the blood are feeding back to the hypothalamus and pituitary, and if fertilization has not occurred the corpus luteum starts to degenerate to a small fibrous patch called the corpus albicans and stops producing progesterone—and menstruation occurs.

If fertilization occurs the corpus luteum keeps on producing progesterone and keeps the thick lining richly supplied with blood for the implanting of the fertilized ovum.

Orgasm is not necessary for fertilization or ovulation or even sexual satisfaction; during intercourse the woman produces mucous secretion from glands at the entrance of the vagina that assist in lubricating the penis. Fertilization usually occurs at or soon after ovulation, but sperm can live for several days. They can be in the Fallopian tubes a few days before ovulation, and several days after ovulation intercourse could result in a sperm making contact with a viable ovum.

In the male the sperm matures in the testes. The process of maturation from a round cell (spermatocyte) to a mobile sperm with a long, powerful tail to project it along takes about two months. The sperm are produced in millions under the influence of hormone from the hypothalamus and pituitary (gonadotrophins) and testicles (testosterone). The sperm pass into the epididymis and up the vas deferens; three glands add secretion to make up the seminal fluid: the prostate, the seminal vesicles, and Cowper's gland. During sexual stimulation the penis greatly enlarges and stiffens and deposits seminal fluid high up in the vagina. This fluid may contain as many as 500 million sperms. If intercourse does not occur, nocturnal emissions dispose of sperm. Masturbation is not necessary or desirable as a method of disposal of old sperm or for relaxation of tension, but it is not harmful. If it becomes a habitual obsessional method of dealing with deliberately aroused sexual desire through self-stimulation then it

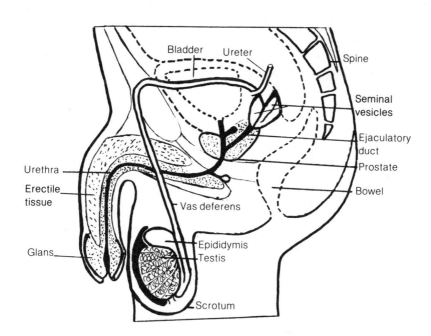

The male reproductive system

is questionable whether it could be harmful to personality development. Many regard this self-centered occupation as quite satisfying. Certainly many married couples when separated from each other find it a means of relieving desire; but this, too, is somewhat different from arousing sexual desire for an unobtainable or forbidden person or directing stimulation to self.

Erection is necessary for intercourse and depends on nerve impulses from the spinal cord that can be affected by higher nerve centers in the brain. Premature ejaculation is a common problem associated with nervous control of sexual feelings. The size of the penis in erection is unrelated to success as a lover and so is its size when not erect, and it is not related to fertility, or to comfort of intercourse. What is essential is that mature sperm are produced in adequate numbers and that the man has patent passages and healthy organs.

Methods of Birth Control

It should now be clear how the male and female reproductive systems can be modified and controlled to reduce or prevent fertilization. It is obvious that obstructing the vas deferens or Fallopian tubes will prevent fertilization. This can occur as the result of venereal disease, and the common method of surgical sterilization is by tying and cutting the passage.

VOLUNTARY STERILIZATION

Voluntary sterilization by vasectomy or tying tubes is becoming an increasingly popular method of birth control with married people who have completed their family, and it is virtually a permanent method: It is very difficult to repair the passage and reverse the operation. It is not a major procedure in either male or female. In most people such operations have no effect on sexual desires or enjoyment, on hormone levels, or on the menstrual cycles; but it must be realized that in the female the ova are released into the abdominal cavity and disintegrate and are absorbed. In the male the only outlet from the testes is closed and the sperms left in the testicle; sperm production is decreased and in some men testosterone production is also decreased. Men are also more likely to have psychological effects than women, particularly if the sexual relationship is not a stable and satisfactory one, and some doubts are now appearing in the medical literature as to its universal desirability. Counseling, careful consideration of all factors, and full acceptance of all the implications by both husband and wife are necessary, and in the majority of people such operations are then successful. But I must admit I shuddered when I read an article in a women's magazine by a wife about "The Wonderful Gift My Husband Gave Me: His Vasectomy."

MECHANICAL METHODS

Mechanical methods of birth control are available for male and female.

The Condom. The condom is a thin rubber sheath pulled over the erect penis, leaving a space at the end to catch the seminal fluid. It is best used with a vaginal lubricant or spermicidal jelly. Condoms are easily available and inexpensive. They put the responsibility on the male and provide the only contraceptive method that offers some protection against venereal disease. There are risks of the condom breaking. It has to be used with care, and it interferes with sensation; but it can be fairly safe used with a spermicidal jelly and, particularly at times when the woman cannot have a reliable method of birth control, it is very acceptable to many people.

The Cervical Diaphragm. More reliable is the rubber cervical diaphragm with a flexible spring around its edge that has to be fitted to be sure of the size. This is inserted by the woman before intercourse, usually with a spermicidal cream; it covers the cervix, so preventing sperm from entering. The woman has to learn how to insert it and usually does so before going to bed and leaves it in place till morning. Both husband and wife are unaware of it during intercourse, and a water douche in the morning makes the method even more reliable. It is a safe, inexpensive method for a responsible woman, but not as completely reliable as methods that suppress ovulation.

Contraceptive Jellies. Chemical methods using contraceptive jellies alone are much less reliable—at best only 90 percent so—but more efficient preparations are being developed and, used in conjunction with the safe period, are reasonably reliable.

PREVENTING IMPLANTATION OF THE FERTILIZED OVUM

The main method is by use of the intrauterine device (IUD). There are several varieties of these and they are inserted into the cavity of the uterus by a doctor; the irritant effect prevents implantation. The IUD tends to increase menstrual bleeding, but it does not otherwise interfere with normal bodily function or desire and it is being used increasingly. It is convenient, there are no pills or appliances that need to be remembered and used effectively, and it can be left in place for a year of more. It may, however, come out, and it is not 100 percent effective, though it is more reliable than most other methods except the hormonal pill. When it has no side effects it is probably the most acceptable method to women. It cannot be used if there is infection or any abnormality of the uterus or if the periods are heavy.

THE PILL

The oral contraceptive pills are of several kinds. All are hormone preparations and they work by preventing ovulation, altering the cervical mucus, and slowing movement down the Fallopian tube. They also alter the lining of the uterus, making implantation less likely.

Use of the pill is more reliable than other methods of contraception because it prevents ovulation and there is no ovum to be fertilized. With it, there is no need for a period of abstinence or for chemical or mechanical methods. However, the pill alters physiological processes and affects every tissue in the body.

There are two main types: (a) a combination of estrogen and progesterone and synthetic preparations made up in varying amounts by different pharmaceutical firms and used for twenty-two days of every cycle; (b) the sequential pills; estrogen for the first two weeks and estrogen and progesterone for the third week. No pill is taken during the fourth week, and with each type withdrawal bleeding occurs. Because the endometrium is less developed, there is less bleeding; and because there is no ovulation and this is not a normal period there are fewer menstrual symptoms. There is also the postcoital pill. A very large dose of estrogen taken within forty-eight hours after intercourse for a period of ten days will also prevent implantation.

Progesterone can be used alone continuously to alter the cervical mucus, but without suppressing ovulation, making it more acceptable to people who wish to preserve ovulation and consider that it should not be suppressed. It can also be used during lactation, wheras the other hormones cannot. Depot progesterone, given as an injection, has an effect that lasts about three months and prevents menstrual bleeding completely.

EFFECTS OF THE PILL

The estrogen-progesterone pills have now been used for more than ten years by millions of women; their full effect will not be known for many years yet. They are effective and safe, in that they present no threat to life, but there are many side effects. For the small percentage of women who are liable to blood changes and thrombosis or clotting they can be dangerous, but low-estrogen pills to a large extent get over this hazard. A recent report from the Royal College of General Practitioners in Britain has been hailed in headlines as exonerating the pill from all criticism. But when one looks at the summarized report as it appeared in the newspapers one sees that while it points to the reliability and convenience and the lessening of symptoms due to normal menstruation (which of course has been removed)—headache, premenstrual depression, abdominal pain at ovulation, excessive bleeding—it still recognizes the small incidence of thrombosis. Temporary and even lengthy sterility occurs, though it mainly responds to further hormone therapy and fertility treatment.

The report seems to contain no evaluation of emotional symptoms or of alteration of sexual desire. Symptoms such as weight gain, skin pigmentation, swollen gums, problems with contact lenses, and nausea may trouble a woman more than they do her doctor; and the personality change that friends and husbands often comment on is not minor to them. Most side effects are said to be removed by changing the pill, and if 99 percent reliability is needed this is the method. It assumes that the pill is taken exactly as directed, for a day missed, a pill not absorbed during a gastric attack or a change in pill without waiting for adjustment can mean pregnancy. There are recent disturbing reports of a slightly increased incidence of serious congenital abnormalities occurring in babies whose mothers continued to take some types of pill before they realized they were pregnant. And there is some evidence that pregnancy occurring in the tubes may be more frequent in women who had previously taken the pill.

It does fill me with some anxiety to contemplate a million nonovulating women caring for children and husbands. And if the pill they are on is one containing a synthetic substance with the action of the male hormone testosterone, what effect may this be having? Some women are quite aggressive enough without a daily dose of male hormone! I am all in favor of birth control and spacing children so that they can receive better care and more love and attention; I deplore the possibility of an overpopulated earth and nothing would please me better than to see women control their own bodies better to improve the success rate of the normal family and the quality of life for all. I am saddened by the disillusionment and obvious unhappiness of the women's liberation extremists and believe that most liberated women, like myself, want to preserve and defend the traditional role of women, want to have their hormones functioning normally or appropriately regulated under medical supervision, and still have the right to work, the right to be individuals.

Natural Methods

The natural methods of avoiding intercourse during the fertile time are becoming increasingly popular and more reliable but are still less reliable than other methods of birth control. They require self-control, periods of abstinence, and the recording of observations, and they depend on accurate recognition of the time of ovulation; they are unlikely to appeal to the irresponsible, the careless, and those who lack self-control. Three methods have been widely used.

The *rhythm method* depends on taking ovulation as the

fourteenth day of the cycle and avoiding intercourse for a week before and after this. It is obviously unreliable when menstruation is irregular, and it makes long periods of abstinence necessary.

The *temperature method* relies on the fact that the body temperature is slightly elevated at ovulation; and after observation of the body temperature over a number of cycles an approximate estimation of ovulation time may be made.

The newest and most reliable method is the *ovulation* or *Billings method*, which relies on the recognition of the nature and amount of the mucous secretion produced around ovulation time and on restricting intercourse to the safe days when there is no secretion, the "dry days." This method will not be practicable for women with cervical or vaginal infections, but normal, healthy ovulating women are well aware of the "mucous symptom" and it has been shown to be a reliable indicator. The ovulation method has the advantages that it reduces the time of abstinence and is applicable during lactation, around the menopause, and for women with irregular periods and no ovum-producing cycles. The mucus is recognizable before ovulation as a slippery secretion that becomes clear and stretchy, and after a woman has observed several cycles she can determine if ovulation is regular and, by recording the mucous symptom, avoid the fertile period; the last day of the mucous symptom is the "peak symptom" and the most likely day of fertilization, and intercourse is avoided for the following four days. Dr. J. and Dr. L. Billings have developed a method of recording the symptom, and research has confirmed its accuracy by determination of hormone levels. It is now widely used by Catholics, and details can be obtained from Catholic family-planning clinics in most cities. The advantages of a method that involves no drugs, no appliances, no cost, and no interference with nature have made it appeal to many young, thinking, responsible people, regardless of religion.

Preventing sperm and ovum from coming into contact at the fertile period can depend on mechanical methods, chemical methods of destroying the sperm, and coitus interruptus. The last-mentioned has been the most widely used method in the world until recently. It is considered unsuitable and psychologically unsatisfactory, but it is still in common use and does not seem to be as disturbing as many people say.

Choosing Which Method

Whatever method of birth control you decide on you should discuss it with a doctor who is interested and experienced in prescribing contraception. It is necessary to find the method that suits the particular couple, so both husband and wife should see the doctor. If the decision is for the diaphragm, IUD, or hormone contraceptive pill, then a thorough examination is necessary and it may well be that several pills may have to be tried. Some doctors will not be prepared to order some methods of contraception. I personally would regard giving hormone contraceptives to teen-age girls as very unsuitable. They are not fully mature, physically or emotionally, not even fully grown, and to deliberately alter the balance of the hypothalamic-pituitary-ovarian axis at this stage seems highly unphysiological. Those who encourage teen-agers in sexual experimentation should remember the increasing venereal disease rate, the rising illegitimacy rate, the higher incidence of cancer of the cervix in sexually experienced teen-agers, their delayed and disturbed emotional development, and their later high marriage-breakdown rate. However, the pill is a risk they should be offered rather than the risk of pregnancy, for it is the safest and most practical method for regular use in the woman who has not borne a child.

Finally, I wonder how many doctors who prescribe the contraceptive pill interview the husbands after a few months of pill usage. In my practice I often see both parents with the child, so I often hear how both sides feel about their sexual relationships. There was an interesting report in the medical literature recently of interviews with the wives of the doctors who were keen on ordering the pill, and a surprising number of their wives were not using that method.

Abortion

What if the contraceptive method fails or you trust to luck and find an unwanted pregnancy on the way? Abortion is now increasingly available and it is not difficult to find a doctor who will do the operation on the grounds of preserving the mental or physical health of the mother, even without a second opinion. It has become the commonest method of birth control. A mother's life and health come first; but I cannot accept abortion performed on demand, or request, as it's euphemistically called. I find a great many women do not know that termination of pregnancy is not a minor operation like a tooth extraction, and that to have an abortion without a very full discussion and assessment of the possible aftereffects is very unwise.

METHODS OF TERMINATION

Aspiration. Aspiration of the contents of the uterus by insertion of a polythene catheter after dilating the os can be done up to eight weeks. It is not always successful and can cause complications. It can miss the products of conception; but it is convenient, since the woman is not usually admitted to a hospital.

Curettage (D and C). Curettage requires anesthesia, dilation of the os, and scraping out of the contents. It is done up to twelve weeks.

Contraction of the Uterine Wall. After twelve weeks methods are used to stimulate the uterine wall to contract and expel the fetus. Prostaglandins have this effect, or saline injected into the uterine cavity. The latter has had many complications and is to be avoided if possible.

Surgical Removal. Surgical removal of the fetus by abdominal operation (doing a mini-Caesarean section) is a more serious procedure and is the method of choice in later pregnancy.

PHYSICAL EFFECTS

The pregnant uterus is soft and richly supplied with blood vessels, and with the best of surgeons under the best of conditions bleeding and perforation of the uterus are common complications, regardless of the method used. Most reports give a 5 percent major complication rate and a 10 percent minor one. Hemorrhage requiring transfusion is the main complication, but just occasionally the bleeding is so severe that the uterus has to be removed to save the woman's life. Infection is not uncommon, and can lead to sterility. The lining of the uterus can be damaged, resulting in disturbance of implantation in future pregnancies and a tendency toward miscarriage or premature birth. This is significant because it endangers the next baby, and there is a higher-than-average incidence of premature babies with problems in subsequent pregnancies of women who have had artificially induced abortions. Some studies of very large numbers give a sterility rate of 5 percent (official Japanese figure, 9 percent) and the sterility does not respond to hormone therapy as does the postpill sterility. The death rate, even with skilled surgery, 9 per 100,000 abortions in Britain, and 8 per 100,000 abortions in New York. These are well-authenticated figures, since abortion is legal and notifiable, and good records are kept.

PSYCHOLOGICAL EFFECTS

Psychological reactions are quite variable, so expert counseling is desirable. The aftereffects may be long-term and not evident until some crisis situation occurs, such as the death of a child or the menopause. Careful evaluation of the situation and sympathetic counseling are essential whether abortion is decided on or not, and it may only be necessary to tide the woman over the first few months of pregnancy, when ambivalent feelings are very common. Abortion is not something to be undertaken lightly; both husband and wife should be involved in the decision, and they should be fully aware of what abortion involves and the possible aftereffects. The risks may be regarded as worth taking in some cases; but for the normal healthy woman who merely wants to delay a pregnancy it may not be advisable.

It is unfortunate that the mass media usually present abortion as a simple procedure that narrow-minded doctors are opposing. This is far from the truth. Those not limited personally by religious beliefs accept abortion as at times necessary and important to the health and happiness of the mother and her family. But the emotional outpourings on TV and in the press make it very difficult for the doctor to make sure that his patient receives the best treatment for *her*. The increase in legal abortions in Britain from 56,000 in 1969 to 127,000 in 1972 (with the introduction of the Abortion Act) and the startling figure of 900,000 abortions in the United States in 1973 seem to imply that the whole matter is being taken very lightly, and that there will be some sad sterile women and some damaged premature babies in the future.

There is no doubt that the earlier the termination is performed, the safer it is for the woman, and if possible this should be within six weeks of conception. However, there are no long-term follow-up figures to evaluate such proved complications as sterility, ectopic pregnancy, subsequent miscarriages, and late psychological effects. After twelve weeks the complications rise sharply.

If an abortion is considered necessary it should be done as soon as possible by a competent, experienced doctor in a hospital, preferably with an overnight stay.

12

Love, Sex, and Marriage

Perhaps a few thoughts on love and human sexuality would be appropriate to end a book on birth and the liberated family. For love, and the sexual attraction between man and woman, created the child; and with the child came the family.

Psychology and Love

As a young enthusiastic pediatrician, determined to learn as much as I could about children and their needs, I wrestled with Freud. While taking a course on Freudian psychology, I was working with a research grant on breast-feeding and I found much that was irreconcilable. Freud's male-dominated psychology, with its lack of understanding of women, made me angry and confused. The professor, a dedicated Freudian, gazed at me with the look of superiority and compassion perfected by many psychiatrists and assured me that he understood my inner thoughts and that all I needed was to be psychoanalyzed. Had I not had a secure and happy marriage, and not found Ian Suttie's *Origins of Love and Hate* and later Erich Fromm's *The Art of Loving* and C. S. Lewis's *Four Loves*, I could have doubted my sanity; and, looking back on this experience, I can well understand women who have not found love becoming savage women's liberationists like Millett and Greer.

As I pursued my search for knowledge about the development of children emotionally and socially, I found D. W. Winnicott, John Bowlby, Arnold Gesell, Rene Spitz, Mary Ainsworth, Melanie Klein, Margaret Ribble, W. Glasser, and many others of a like mind, who cared about children. Books like *Determinants of Infant Behaviour* and other similar composite works have somehow woven together reality and fantasy for me. Freud has fallen into perspective; and his daughter, Anna, following his work, has clarified it and added a woman's touch.

Prominent in all this work is the theme of *caring concern*, a term much more explicit than *love*. After Freud and the psychoanalytic schools of psychology came the various behaviorist psychologists and "behavior modification." More recently still came the "encounter groups," which can be so dangerous when they separate caring concern and causation from techniques and manipulation of human emotions. One of the most damaging experiences for any young person is to have emotional reactions manipulated. I know a lovely, intelligent college student who was seduced by her philosophy professor into her first sexual intercourse on the argument that this was a valuable experience, that she must learn the techniques of sex and be able to enjoy all varieties of sexual and sensual experience without being emotionally involved. She, poor child, at seventeen thinks he is wonderful and that he really cares for her, even as he tells her that he is teaching other girls this same valuable lack of sensitivity and avoidance of lasting involvement.

The lack of caring concern of some of these manipulators is quite terrifying. To be in an encounter group and be told by a self-satisfied philosopher to hold the hands of a stranger, gaze into her eyes, and tell her something about your sex life that you have never told anybody before (as occurred in a family-life seminar) makes one realize the total lack in such people of responsibility and sensitivity, of respect for privacy and integrity. Used wisely, the encounter group can be an enriching experience, as some marriage counselors are finding. Better still are the "growth groups" of Professor Clinebell. People can learn a great deal about each other and communicate their feelings with the guidance of a leader concerned with their welfare; but if unqualified and unethical people use these techniques their discussion, get-together, and touch groups can have very different results. The groups can become stroking, sensation-stimulating parties, in which the participants try to recapture the sensations they should have received as babies—when their sensation receptors were also those of babies.

I recently heard a senior social worker expressing anxiety at the lack of sensitivity, the lack of appreciation of the need for confidentiality and trust, in some of the young social workers coming into her department. She wondered if the encounter-groups training they were receiving could be responsible. It can be good to have one's emotions stirred and to understand their origins; but stir them too frequently and they become dulled. It is also devastating and criminal to leave people with their defenses torn down, exposed to public view, and feeling worthless and unloved. All groups should be under the supervision of well-trained people and one must know the philosophy of the group leader.

Everyone who has ever loved, and every primitive community and civilization that recognizes love, accepts the essential components of love as faith, trust, loyalty, concern for the welfare of the loved one, willingness to meet his needs—and a belief that this loving concern will last.

Sexual Attraction

Sex is a biological urge that is essential for the reproduction of the race. Man is easily aroused and has only to contribute his seed; woman, having to nurture the child that may result, needs love and a lasting relationship. We are well aware that both men and women can learn the techniques of sexual stimulation to orgasm and find great pleasure in sex as a recreation; and we know that sex can be used as a profession. But this is not love. Procreational sex need not include love; recreational sex excludes love. Love requires a lasting relationship.

The idealistic humanist, James Hemming, says that "personal fulfillment is attainable only through the implementation of certain principles. One is that it is not possible in sexual relationships to be both *casual* and *deep*. . . . Herein lies the frustration of the Casanovas and the nymphomaniacs. Such people behave as though sexual satisfaction lies in the quantity of experience, whereas it lies in the quality of experience." It is

surprising that Hemming, while recognizing the depth and ex-
clusiveness of this most satisfying of all love relationships, can
think that lifting strictures on premarital sexual relationships will
make marriage-partner selection more successful. Many studies
have shown that premarital intercourse does not assist sexual
adjustment in marriage; in fact, it correlates with extramarital sex
later (Kinsey, Wilson, in an American Institute of Family
Relations study). In approving taking and experiencing without
acquiring self-control and self-discipline and developing loyalty
and understanding of the needs of one another, Hemming fails to
appreciate how the physical excitement takes over and what the
difference is between the emotions of men and women. The
immature adolescent, confusing love with biological urges and
searching for instant sexual ecstasy, is likely to be hurt. The girl,
particularly, is left feeling used, disillusioned, and will be uncertain in her next sexual adventure; and if that does not lead to
marriage she is likely to continue in superficial relationships.

In the report of a seminar held by the Society of Medical
Psychoanalysts in New York in March 1973 there were several
interesting papers on "The Effects of Adolescent Sexual Experience," all of which reported that sexual intercourse in young
and mid-adolescent girls was damaging to ego development and
self-identification. "Mature love was not possible and involvement in sexual intercourse diverted the adolescent from the
major tasks of the age period." Halleck, observing students on
campus and then reporting the experience of psychiatrists,
suggests that the ability to form lasting relationships may be
affected also in older students who become involved with multiple
partners. "The student psychiatrists see more and more recently
married couples who find themselves unable to tolerate the
possibility of loving one person intimately or remaining faithful to
that person. . . . The new era of promiscuity seems to have done
little to enhance the female student's image of herself as a
productive and responsible person."

Somehow every man and woman in the street knows what
happens to girls who have been involved in numerous sexual
relationships: No one regards them as good mother material or as
good marriage risks. Michael Schofield's report on adolescent
behavior confirms this. Only the disillusioned humanist who has

lost her ideals and is usually divorced wants to see her daughter involved in premarital sex; yet there are academics (mostly psychologists and philosophers), a few abortionist and humanist doctors, and the pornography pushers, who want to encourage adolescents and even preadolescents in sexual experimentation and in deviant practices. They approve premarital intercourse, petting to orgasm in casual relationships, habitual masturbation; and some even believe sodomy and fellatio and bestiality to be harmless and appropriate experience for the teen-ager. Obviously they accept that abortion should be available to all on request, but they rarely talk about its risks.

Love and Marriage

In advocating the sexual relationship that is to the exclusion of all others, and the importance of maturity and self-discipline in this relationship, it must not be thought that I undervalue the techniques of sexuality. For the man and woman committed to each other, the involvement of the total person, the synchronizing of desire, can reach heights of enjoyment possible only with practice and skillful, sensitive, expert techniques. For too many people, sex has been shrouded in romantic mystery or an aura of shameful sin, and the Kinseys, and Masters and Johnson, have at least torn off the shrouds and revealed pleasure and excitement even in "sex without passion"—that poor degrading shadow of the real thing.

Better understanding of sexuality has improved technique for many who had inhibitions about their sex feelings and has enabled them to communicate more effectively. Satisfying sexual performance cannot be taken as the unfailing criterion of a happy marriage, and it is important to distinguish between competent sexual performance and total personal involvement.

My extensive search of the literature has found no valid scientific evidence to support the contention of the proponents of the permissive society that premarital and extramarital sexual intercourse in adolescence, or even later, is other than destructive to personality development and the fully satisfying sexual relationship. One wades through Alex Comfort and the sexology magazines in search of reputable studies in psychology, philosophy, sociology, and medical science—all to no avail. In fact, as one studies the material produced by SIECUS,* much of it very well produced and useful, one cannot fail to become anxious about Dr. Mary Calderone's lack of appreciation of the young child's sensitivity needs, about the involvement of such leading SIECUS authorities as Isodore Rubin and Kirkendall in commercial sexology, and about SIECUS condoning Albert Ellis for "uninvolved sex."

Oftentimes, these proponents of "uninvolved sex" are as deficient in their knowledge of female psychology as they are in scientific logic. In defense of the contraceptive pill, they insist that the mortality of pregnancy is much greater than that of the pill. What they fail to point out is that pregnancy results in a baby and a new life is commenced. Furthermore, the pregnancy mortality figures include those of women with many varieties of serious illness who are prepared to risk their lives because they so desperately want a child, and they also include the deaths from abortion. To translate this situation into an argument for encouraging adolescents to use contraceptives and have early sexual intercourse is, to say the least, unscientific. Those who belong to the "as long as nobody gets hurt" school of thought fail to realize that poor little Miss Nobody is too much a nobody for many men to realize that she is being hurt, and that adolescents are not mature enough to make irreversible decisions that can seriously affect their future.

The last two decades have seen women rebel, rightly, against male-dominated attitudes toward sex and against the dual standard; there has been a great obsession with sex techniques and sex deviation; and there has been an increase in sexual experience at a casual and noninvolved level in younger and younger age groups. Many women have seen the adoption of the male standard as liberation. Pitirim Sorokin says, "Increasing divorce and desertion and the growth of prenuptial and extramarital sex relations are signs of sex addiction somewhat similar to drug addiction." Pornography has become the drug of the sex-obsessed and, as with all addictive drugs, there are degrees of involvement. There are the samplers who see no harm in it. There are those who

*Sex Information and Education Council of the United States.

become addicted and try to involve others in their addiction. There are those who make money out of it as the pushers and manufacturers. The pushers of pornography often have the mass media and big money at their disposal and they profess to be espousing the cause of liberty.

Influencing Children

Our children are going to be exposed to sexually explicit and sexually deviant material, and they are also going to be influenced by some teachers and colleagues who accept or propound permissive philosophies. The subject of sex education in schools will at times be in the hands of teachers who, perhaps to justify their own sexual practices, teach sex education without moral values. They see themselves as enlightened, when in fact they are usually unloved: They wish to destroy the family pattern that gave them so little. The child may see only an attractive young teacher apparently enjoying sexual license. He cannot see the future or the past of such a person or the amazing epidemics of venereal disease and pubic lice and scabies that have involved millions of people in the United States, despite improved hygiene and tremendous advances in treatment.

The statistics for abortion and births to unmarried mothers are available, but their full significance is lost on a child. His only protections are that he should learn the meaning of love and the family at home and that his parents should become involved in what he is taught at school.

It seems from many studies that a stable society depends on the majority of the people having a stable home life, and that the disruptive elements in our society come in general from homes with insufficient or inadequate expression of love. If only a fraction of the money spent on going to the moon or on preparation for war could be spent on preparation for marriage, family life, and childbirth, on teaching people the meaning of love and the joy of lasting human relationships! If only we could stop studying evil and tragedy and study the factors that make for happiness, what a change there could be in the world!

Why is such a wonderful and all-pervading medium as television, which could bring so much happiness, inspiration, and beauty into our homes, bringing so much violence and transitory sex and giving such a false image to young people of what a full life means? Now that TV, radio, beautifully produced magazines, and all forms of education, come direct to our children, bypassing the parents even in early infancy, those who care what happens to children must take a more active interest in the messages they are receiving. We cannot, indeed must not, exclude the technical wonders, but we can influence the way they are being used. Our family circle is too fragile these days for us to ignore the pressures that are on it.

Parent Power, Sex Education, and Moral Values

In an affluent materialistic society, so many are grabbing what they can—the second job with cash payment to avoid paying taxes, for instance. The shoplifting figures show even more dishonesty in this area than in the sexual field; there is an increase in violent crime, in stealing, in greed; the search for sensationalism and excitement seems to have people saying, "Am I missing something? Have I got all I can get?" There is a frightening lack of concern about the personal welfare of others. Throw them some money, but care what happens to them? No!

Could the answer lie in what we parents are putting into life? *We* care what happens to *our* children. But do we care enough to demand that neither our children nor journalists, nor actors and actresses, be exploited by the money-makers who seem bent on trying to change our family way of life? Confused parents, dazzled by change, more than a little envious of their children's freedom, and awed by the educators, still care about their own children. Can Parent Power help children, or are parents too apathetic, too selfish, or too unsure of their own standards and security?

In teaching the adolescent about sexuality it is essential—if he is to choose the lifetime partner needed to rear children successfully—to present as the ideal the most satisfying that can be achieved: the lasting man-woman relationship. The adolescent has a right to be helped to learn to distinguish the factors that can destroy or seriously endanger the possibility of his achieving that ideal. Two such factors are physical involvement in homosexual practices and promiscuity in adolescence. Any education program in sexuality must be fully oriented to help the teen-ager delay his decisions on involvement in sexual intercourse until he is an adult. He or she is then in a better position to accept the heterosexual long-term commitment needed for family life, or to decide to sublimate sexual energy in career and friendships, or adopt the life of casual heterosexual relationships or homosexuality (in either case, one hopes, giving up the idea of rearing children).

Was mathematics ever satisfactorily taught by showing children how to get the wrong answers? Education in human sexuality should aim to show the happiest and most satisfactory way of rearing the next generation. One learns love by seeing and taking part in successful relationships, and by starting at birth. The famous Russian educator of the Revolution, Makarenko, almost Russia's counterpart of Spock, says in his *Book for Parents,* "Teaching young people to love, teaching them to know love, teaching them to be happy means teaching them self-respect and human dignity. No educational trips into the autonomous republic of Venus will help you there. In human society, especially in socialist society, sex education cannot be physiological education. The sexual act cannot be isolated from all the achievements of human culture, from the conditions of life and man in society, from the humanitarian course of history, from the triumphs of aesthetics."

An extract from the Soviet monthly *Journal of the Academy of Educational Sciences* is also of interest:

"In October 1917 socialist revolution wiped out the political, legal and economic inequality of women, but some people have incorrectly understood this freedom and have decided that human sex life can be carried out with a disorderly succession of husbands and wives. In a tightly organized society, a socialist's society, such practices necessarily lead to laxity and vulgarization of relationships unworthy of man, cause difficult personality problems, unhappiness and disruption of the family making orphans of the children.

"Every parent must work toward training the future citizen to be happy only in family love and to seek the joys of sex life only in marriage. If parents do not set such a goal for themselves and do not reach it, their children will lead a promiscuous sex life full of dramas, unhappiness, misery and injury to society."

There certainly are some leftists or Communists in our own society who have not yet caught up with the change in Soviet policy. In fact, some of the literature on sex education with well-know Communist names in its authorship would have some trouble getting into Russia; and I wonder what these propagandist authors would think of Russia's compulsory three months' engagement period?

The child learns attitudes to sex in his own home. In the early years his parents answer his questions as they arise, and the child learns how men and women treat each other by seeing his mother and father talking and living together.

Sex education in the primary school needs the full participation of parents in parent-child sessions, with films and educational material. The child is entitled to the physical facts, but in this period of latent sexuality stimulation of sexual emotions is better delayed. Educational programs by teachers or doctors can be presented at the late primary or secondary school stage to complete the parents' work and fill the gaps. Parents are entitled to protect their children against being indoctrinated with philosophies that oppose their way of life. They are entitled to know what is in any program on human relationships that is planned, and to be aware of the philosophy of the teacher in charge of it.

What of Love?

The philosopher Schwarz says, "Love is perpetual striving, unending uncertainty and insecurity, an everlasting act of creation." I prefer Erich Fromm, who says, "Love is the only rational answer to the problem of human existence. . . . Love is an act of faith and whoever is of little faith is also of little love. . . . It requires the development of humility, objectivity and reason." Suttie believes that the requirements of love are "company, awareness of each other's needs and acceptance of certain moral standards. . . . Morals are not religious beliefs, morals are the standards of behavior that enable people to live together in a society, caring for each other, recognizing each other's welfare as necessary to preserve the society, acceptance of responsibility for each other."

The family that is the basic unit of our society is now a man, his wife, and their children. It can be "an everlasting act of creation," growing as it meets the needs of all its members; it can be the most exciting and fulfilling experience that anyone can have. Fromm says it must include "respect for all its members, self-respect in all, knowledge of each and response to each other's needs." This is caring concern. Surely Fromm's approach is humanism at its best and comes very near to but is not quite the same as the Christian ethic of loving others as oneself, giving not taking, recognizing the need for personal integrity, moral standards, the rights of the individual, and the sanctity of life. Suttie is realistic when he says love needs company. I am surprised at how many men have breakfast alone and even make their own lunches and sometimes the children's too.

(I do like my cup of tea in bed in the morning; but surely a man is entitled to his wife's company at breakfast, even if she is not at her best conversationally or pictorially. My mother brought us up to regard breakfast as a very important meal nutritionally; no toast and coffee for us: good Scottish porridge and bacon and eggs; but then she was English and my father was Scottish. Naturally, I have been influenced by this background, but I still believe that good food and good company make a good way to start the day.)

This love that brings man and woman together, that fulfills the sexual urge and the need for a lasting relationship and has a stake in the future with a child to nurture—it needs communication, variety, continual refreshment, and laughter together. Let there be a night away from the children, a little more attention to the art of lovemaking—technique is important—special occasions to recapture the falling-in-love days and revive the physical attraction, special participation in mutual interests. Life can become so serious when dominated by the twenty-four-hour responsibility of children, and the need to work for life's necessities and a confusing array of luxuries. Burdened by duties and by routine, many think that they have lost romance and even erotic pleasure, and they are tempted into extramarital relationships and the escapist fantasy world of those who mistake sensuality for love. This can be catastrophic if they realize their mistake too late to save their marriage, or if they enter on the endless search for more and more exciting sensation—only to find that they have destroyed their personal integrity as well as the happiness of those they loved. The love I speak of can resist that blinding flash of sexual attraction to which many succumb and which usually passes.

Our children learn from us by imitation. If you don't believe me, then watch your four-year-old daughter playing with her dolls or a group playing mothers and fathers. Failure to develop a good working love relationship in the marriage will hurt the child throughout life. Isn't it worth a lot of study, discussion, and communication to develop and preserve it?

Most marriages do not break down primarily because of sexual problems but because of failures in human relationships and everyday living; and it is usually the man who will not take part in marriage guidance, which can improve communication and awareness of needs and technique. He tends to see marriage guidance as a threat to his masculinity rather than as a way of improving relationships. Separation or divorce, with a man having access to his child for one day a week, does not show the child a father in action; it shows him a man who has failed to make his marriage work and it may teach him that running away from a difficult situation can appear to be a satisfactory solution. Many men, I realize, are in the situation of the old man who left home and on being reproached by the priest for deserting his wife said, "Father, I'm no deserter, I'm a refugee!" and my comments on reconciliation and facing responsibility refer equally to women.

You have a child who is part of you both, a child who loves and needs you both. You suffer with him, you rejoice with him, you try to drag him back from danger, and you try to push him forward to test his ability. An emotionally disturbed child becomes an emotionally disturbed parent; his emotional development is in your hands. You are parents with equal responsibility for protecting and rearing the child to maturity; you are now involved in a new love. You may have been un-fortunate in the quality of parental love you received and in what you believe society did to you, and you may be insecure and find it difficult to express what you feel. You may find, as you talk to your parents now that *they* did not express what they felt very well.

Love is an art that is learned. You can love a baby; you can nurture the love between you that gave him life. Fromm says, "The deepest need of man is to overcome his separateness. Love is union under the conditions of preserving one's integrity." The theologians say the same thing but they get very mixed up with the don'ts and sometimes forget the do's. The liberated family is united with love in the ascendant despite frictions. Each member has individuality and integrity. Human rights, woman's rights, the rights of the child, all cease to be something to be fought for and demanded in this environment and become something readily given with love and understanding. Idealistic? Yes. But impossible? No.

No one expects to live always on the mountaintops: We have to descend into the marketplace and even the valleys to strengthen relationships. One has to feel jealousy and isolation to know the reality of love. The breaking up of many marriages could have been avoided if only the partners had shut out the rest of the world for a while and thought about each other.

Where is the hope for the future? We have a sick society, undisciplined and self-centered, but it need not destroy itself and die as so many civilizations have before. We have the knowledge to cure our sick society, and the medicine; but the treatment needed is drastic. Though governments can make plans and laws, our cure cannot be administered by government edict; it takes individuals to achieve this.

I hope that there will be changes in our doctor/nurse-centered maternity hospitals to improve conditions for the beginning of life; I hope that education for family life will set moral standards in schools; I hope that health education will become an essential and accepted part of hospital care. I hope that the community will realize that no society should allow the unborn to be killed just because a woman finds it inconvenient to be pregnant. The increase in abortions in countries where abortion has been legalized and paid for from public funds has shown that therapeutic abortion has been extended to abortion on demand. If the law is thus to determine what is right and wrong for the average citizen, it must surely remain stricter where life is concerned, or how long will it be before the aged and the handicapped who are economic burdens on society will follow the unborn child and be destroyed by the selfish and the irresponsible for trivial reasons? Where then is tenderness and compassion? Where is concern for our fellows? Having seen how Hitler set out to exterminate the Jews and the mentally handicapped, surely we have now learned that every individual has personal responsibility for what happens to other people and particularly to his children.

We now have methods of improving the quality of life. We can prevent many congenital abnormalities; genetic counseling is improving; population control is possible; family life can be strengthened to provide the best conditions for rearing children. If the family is a bad family that is self-destructive and damaging the children, it should be disbanded. It is better to have one responsible parent than two unhappy ones, and better to have none than two irresponsible ones when the state can provide foster parents or adoptive parents. We need more facilities for taking early measures to prevent marriage breakdown; and we need better means of terminating the failed marriage with justice, but less traumatically and less expensively. There will always be those who cannot achieve the long-term harmonizing of two personalities that make the satisfying marriage; there will be some who make their marriage relationship so exclusive that even the children feel shut out; there will be many who make the best of an imperfect situation; and there will be those who find other ways of expressing their love.

This book is for those who are planning a family and must now think of the child's future as well as their own. They must build a better world for him, a world that shows compassion and tenderness for those damaged by society and recognizes that the best way to prevent damage to future children is to strengthen the family. To me this means a rejection of the philosophies that hold human life lightly and preach self-gratification and the don't-get-involved-in-depth way of life. As a Christian, I worship a God of love, and though I am disturbed at what is done in his name, my experience and my scientific knowledge tell me that the basic truths about life lie in his teaching regardless of what man does with it.

For the sake of the children, parents must get involved. If the predators and exploiters are not controlled and our children are not taught responsibility, caring concern for others, and self-control, then the future is bleak. The last word on marriage I leave to Dr. Robert H. Williams, in his book *To Live and to Die: When, Why, and How.*

"In our modern world where the individual feels lost in the human throng, the desire for real personal involvement—relationship in depth—is greater now than ever before. The prevailing malaise of our era lies in our rootlessness, isolation, and loss of identity. Only the experience of being a significant part of the life of another can cure this condition. Regardless of the many alternatives proposed by the critics of marriage, marriage uniquely offers a deep and lasting relationship of openness, trust, and sharing with a loved person. Marriage fulfills much of what we seek as we drift through life, hoping and being disappointed by superficial relationships. On the other hand, many marriages have caused great unhappiness, causing failure in social and business relationships, failure of mental and physical health, suicide, and homicide. . . . The dividends of marriage depend considerably on the extent to which we invest in its success."

Appendix 1:
Prenatal Exercises

Many hospitals offer expectant parents a preparation-for-childbirth program. The aim is to tell *both* parents something of the principles of mother and child care. Lecture demonstrations are held in the evenings, when expectant fathers can also attend. Films are shown and various aspects of parentcraft are discussed.

Morning classes are held in the physiotherapy department for the expectant mother where she is given detailed instruction in baby care and preparing herself for birth.

The exercises, controlled relaxation, and breathing techniques shown on this page serve as a reminder for the daily routine at home and do not replace attendance at classes. The daily practice of this routine, together with a clear understanding of your part in labor, is wise preparation for childbirth.

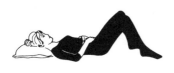

To help keep your abdominal muscles in trim during pregnancy: Lie on your back with knees bent up, feet on the floor. Without raising your chest, tighten abdominal muscles slowly and firmly. Relax.

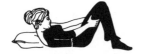

To help with a labor room position: Lift head and shoulders off pillow, tucking hands behind knees. Relax

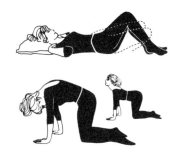

To keep your lower spine flexible during pregnancy: Keeping shoulders firmly on the floor, swing knees first to the right, then to the left, rhythmically.

Another exercise to relieve backache during pregnancy: Kneel on hands and knees; drop head down, rounding back; then raise head, and relax back.

To help with bladder control during pregnancy contractions: Tighten muscles around front and back passages, drawing up pelvic floor. Relax.

An exercise for the labor room: Hold your breath, push down gently, relaxing your pelvic floor. Practice this "push and let it come" for the second stage, once only each day. Not to be done in the last six weeks.

CONTROLLED RELAXATION

Your role during dilation contractions is to relax and "let go" with each one. This needs daily practice since relaxation during labor is *not* easy. Practice this exercise lying on your side, and also lying on your back.

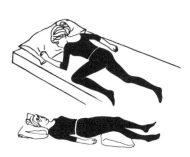

Tense up as you have been taught. Then "let go" all over, breathe deeply and slowly, feeling limp and heavy. Become familiar with the difference between "tensing up" and relaxing. Tension is tiring, and it interferes with the normal pattern of labor; relaxation allows the uterus to work efficiently. Remember that relaxation is your aim through each dilation contraction.

BREATHING EXERCISES TO HELP
WITH BREATHING CONTROL DURING LABOR

1. Relaxation breathing for dilation contractions. With open mouth or through your nose practice deep rhythmical breathing with long breaths out—"sighing-breathing"—to help you with your relaxation.
2. Panting-breathing—if you are asked to stop pushing. With open mouth, take a number of quick shallow breaths. This creates a panting

effect. Practice this rhythmic panting. Remember this "in-case-you-need-it" breathing is never used for relaxation but is a help in overcoming the urge to push at the end of the first stage and delivery.

3. "Bearing-down" breathing for pushing contractions. With open mouth, take one deep breath and hold it as long as you can. Then let that breath out, take another, and hold it again. Repeat a third time.

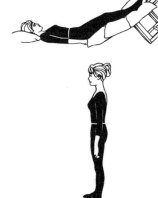

ACHING LEGS?

Rest with legs elevated on upturned chair as you have been shown.

POSTURE

Stand tall but comfortably, with shoulders relaxed. Remember to ease the curve in your lower back, keeping your pelvis tucked underneath your baby.

BREATHING TECHNIQUES TO HELP
DURING CHILDBIRTH

1. *Ordinary* normal, quiet breathing, deliberately relaxing in standing, sitting, or lying down during *early* labor contractions.
2. When relaxation becomes difficult during strengthening contractions, *deep, slow, sighing-breathing* helps relaxation during a contraction. Ordinary, normal breathing, resting in between contractions.
3. *Mask* breathing. Breathe through your *mouth.* Start right at the beginning of the contraction. Press mask firmly into your face. Faster, deep breathing. Ordinary breathing, resting in between contractions. No mask.
4. *Panting-breathing* if you are asked to use this at end of the first stage of labor, when you have a contraction. It will not take away the *urge* to push, but helps you *not* to push on an undilated cervix.
5. *Hold breath* to push efficiently with expulsive second-stage contractions.
6. *Pant (shallow) or push,* as told by doctor, for delivery of the baby's head and body.

Appendix 2:
Postnatal Exercises

Now you've had your baby, it is important to do a few simple exercises to improve the tone of muscles stretched during pregnancy and baby's birth. It is well worthwhile doing them daily, about six times each, for two or three months after leaving the hospital. They have been kept to a minimum to fit in with a busy routine.

1. *Pelvic floor contractions:* Tighten and draw in strongly the muscles around your front and back passages, as if trying to prevent yourself from passing water and having a bowel action. Relax slowly. Repeat often during the day. Do this exercise also when standing and sitting.

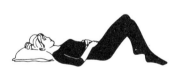

2. *For abdominal muscles:* Without raising your chest, draw in abdominal muscles really firmly. Hold to a count of six. Relax slowly. Repeat often during the day. Do this exercise also when standing and sitting.

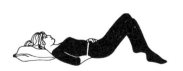

3. Pelvic control: Place one hand in the small of your back, and the other on your abdomen. Draw in abdominal muscles and at the same time flatten the small of your back. Then draw up

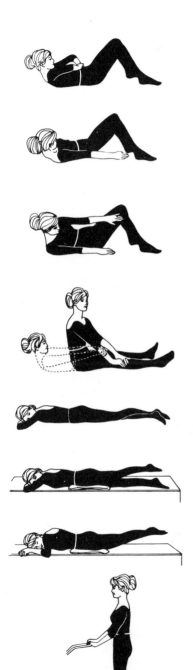

pelvic floor muscles as in 1. Relax slowly. This can be done standing or sitting, whenever you think of it.

4. *For a trim waist:* Hands on lower abdomen, draw in abdominal muscles. Raise head, shoulders, and elbows from bed, keeping chin tucked in. Lower slowly.

. *To progress this exercise:* Tighten abdominal muscles, lift head so that chin is on your chest, then reach down with right hand to touch right ankle. Repeat to opposite side.

5. *For abdominal muscles:* Tighten abdominal muscles, then reach left hand across to outside of right knee, lifting head and left shoulder as you come. Relax and repeat to opposite side.

To progress this exercise: Knees straight, roll up slowly to the sitting position, reaching both hands toward left knee. Unroll *slowly* back to lying. Repeat to opposite side.

6. *Pelvic floor control:* Lie face down, with legs crossed. Squeeze thighs together, tighten up inside, tense from hips to toes. Relax slowly.

7. *Back-strengthening exercise:* With a pillow under your pelvis, lie face down and, keeping knees straight, lift alternate legs just clear of the bed. Lower slowly.

To progress this exercise: Lift both legs together (knees straight) and lower slowly.

Don't be a gone-in-the-middle, round-shouldered mother! Remember to stand "tall" but comfortably, straightening out the curve in your lower back.

Glossary

Abortion The termination of pregnancy either spontaneously or by medical or surgical means, after implantation and before the child is viable, now interpreted as twenty weeks.

Adrenal glands Ductless endocrine glands situated on the upper surface of each kidney. Each gland consists of two parts: a cortex that produces corticosteroids concerned with body metabolism, particularly mineral fluid and glucose; and a medulla that secretes adrenalin, which stimulates the sympathetic nervous system, the part of the nervous system concerned with fight and flight.

Afterbirth The placenta, the structure through which the developing child is nourished.

Amnion The inner of the two membranes that contain amniotic fluid and the developing child, the "bag of waters."

Antenatal Time from conception to the birth of the baby, now more often known as prenatal, probably because many people misspell the word as antinatal.

Anus External opening of the lower bowel, back passage.

Areola Dark area surrounding the nipple under which lie the lacteal sinuses.

Breech birth When the baby appears tail first; not as safe as head first, the usual way.

Carbohydrates Organic compounds of which starches and sugars are important ingredients, providing about 50 percent of the calories for most people's diet, and roughage as cellulose.

Castration Removal of gonads (i.e., testis or ovary) that produce the sperm and ova essential for reproduction.

Cervix Neck of uterus.

Chorion Outer of the two membranes surrounding the amniotic fluid and developing child.

Chromosomes Rod-shaped bodies in the nucleus of every cell in the body, arranged in identically shaped pairs, one from each parent, but with different genetic material in the genes that have fixed positions along the chromosome and supply the inherited characteristics. Chromosomal abnormalities produce serious congenital abnormalities.

Circumcision Surgical removal of the foreskin, a protective flap of tissue protecting the glans of the penis from irritation. The foreskin cannot normally be pulled back to show the glans until the baby is several months old, but is usually retractable before two years. The operation is nonessential but occasionally indicated and often requested for religious or hygienic reasons.

Clitoris Part of the female external genitalia, a small very sensitive organ about one inch in front of the external opening of the bladder. It becomes swollen and erect during intercourse and is concerned with the sensation of orgasm.

Coitus Sexual intercourse, copulation, between male and female, with penis entering the vagina.

Colostrum Fluid secreted in the breast before the true milk comes in. It is present during the last months of pregnancy and during the first few days after the birth of the baby. Only a few milliliters can be expressed at a time, but it is rich in protein that protects against infection, particularly viral infection.

Condom Rubber sheath used as contraceptive to cover the penis and catch spermatic fluid.

Cross-matching In giving blood transfusions it is essential that the blood of the patient and the donor are compatible. Mainly this depends on the blood group to which they belong, but before commencing a transfusion some of the patient's blood and the blood to be used in the transfusion are mixed to make sure that clotting together of the cells does not occur. This is known as cross-matching.

Curette   Instrument used to scrape out the products of conception in surgical abortion.

DNA   Deoxyribonucleic acid, a chemical substance making up the genes in the nucleus of all cells.

Diaphragm   A partition separating two surfaces: e.g., the large muscle separating the chest and abdomen and responsible for about 60 percent of respiratory effort. The rubber cap with a spring in the outer ring that is used to cover the cervix during intercourse as a contraceptive device.

Diuretic   A chemical substance used as medication to increase the output of urine and remove fluid that has been accumulating in the tissues.

Douche   A vaginal washout, usually administered with a can and tube, with the tube inserted into the vagina and the can elevated sufficiently for the fluid to flow freely into and out of the vagina. It is important that the fluid is not introduced under pressure.

Dysmature fetus   When the baby developing in the uterus appears to be smaller than expected it may be failing to thrive from poor nutrition or ill health. A baby born at term but smaller than average is regarded as dysmature and requires special care.

Ectoderm   One of the three primitive embryonic layers of tissue from which the body grows. From it develop skin, brain, hair, nails, nerves, and organs of sensation.

Edema   Swelling of tissues.

Ejaculation   Expulsion of seminal fluid during a climax of sexual intercourse in the male.

Embryo   The developing child from implantation to twelve weeks.

Endoderm   One of the three primitive layers in the embryo from which the child develops. It provides most of the internal organs.

Endometrium   Cells lining the uterus. The thickness of the layer varies according to hormonal stimulation. The endometrium is discharged during menstruation and renewed during the month.

Enema   Bowel washout, usually done after labor has commenced to ensure that the passage through the pelvis is as clear as possible for the baby.

Epididymis   Cordlike structure that can be felt along the side of the testis that stores sperms.

Episiotomy   A cut made at the external outlet of the vagina to allow easier passage of the baby during birth or to avoid a tear in a damaging place. Usually done in breech, forceps, and premature deliveries.

Erection   The tissue in the penis fills with blood on sexual excitement and causes the penis to become firm and erect and capable of entry into the vagina.

Estrogen   Female sex hormone. There are now synthetically produced chemical substances widely used to produce similar effects.

Exchange transfusion   The process whereby the blood in the body is largely removed and replaced with blood from another person. This is done by removing about 10 ml. at a time and injecting 10 ml. It is a long and tedious process, not without risk, and should be done by doctors familiar with the technique. It is used for babies with severe jaundice, usually due to Rh incompatibility or prematurity, and also in some cases of poisoning.

Fallopian tube   The tube through which the ovum passes to reach the uterus. If it is blocked by past venereal infection or abnormality pregnancy cannot occur without treatment.

Fecal softener   Medication to ensure that the feces do not become hard and painful to pass.

Feces   Contents of the lower bowel.

Fetus   Developing child from twelve weeks to time of birth.

Fontanel   The diamond-shaped area of the top of the head in the baby where the frontal and parietal bones meet. It allows skull growth and remains open until well into the second year; "the soft spot."

Forceps   Surgical instrument consisting of two blades shaped to fit the head of the baby, one being slipped down each side of the head and traction applied during contractions to assist in the delivery of the baby if the mother is not making adequate progress or the baby is becoming distressed.

Frontal bone   That part of the skull that makes the forehead.

Fundus   Upper part of the uterus.

Genes   Ultramicroscopic particles that carry the hereditary material arranged in pairs along the chromosomes.

Gestation   Pregnancy.

Gonad   Testis, ovary.

Gonorrhea   The commonest venereal disease in male and female, it spreads up the reproductive organs infecting the lining of cervix and tubes in the female and the urethra, prostate, and epididymis in the male. It may cause sterility and is often not recognized in the female. It is a notifiable disease and is becoming more resistant to treatment. (Infecting organism: gonococcus.)

Gynecologist   A physician who specializes in the treatment of diseases of the female reproductive organs.

Heterosexuals   Persons whose sexual desires are directed toward persons of the opposite sex. All societies exercise some control over heterosexual physical activity in the interests of the community, and those who sublimate their sexual energy and direct it into other channels are not abnormal or damaging themselves.

Homosexual   A person whose sexual desires are directed toward persons of the same sex. A distinction is usually made between those physically involved in homosexual practices and those who direct their sexual energy by sublimation into other activities.

Hormones   Chemical substances secreted by the endocrine ductless glands and passed into the bloodstream, having specific effects on different organs.

Husband   It seems absurd to have to define the term, but a husband is a man who has committed himself legally to one woman with the intention of establishing a lifetime relationship with her for love and companionship, and usually with the intention of rearing a family and establishing a home.

Hydramnios   Excessive accumulation of amniotic fluid surrounding the developing child. It may occur with twins and be associated with premature births, with some abnormal conditions of the child, and with retention of fluid in the mother's tissues.

Hypertension   Rise in blood pressure. It may occur during pregnancy and is one of the main risks that doctors carefully observe. It can be successfully treated and is dangerous untreated.

Hypothalamus   The part of the brain that is vitally concerned with the endocrine glands, forming releasing substances that set off hormone production and receiving feedback from all endocrine glands and stimulation from higher brain centers. It is virtually the regulating mechanism for the endocrine system.

Hysterectomy   Removal of the uterus by surgery.

Impotence   Inability of the male to carry out the sexual act, usually due to failure of erection or inability to maintain an erection.

Induction of labor   Artifical commencement of labor by medical or surgical means. Synthetic oxytocin drip into the bloodstream stimulates the uterus to contract; rupture of the membranes releases some amniotic fluid, and change in pressure causes the uterus to start to contract. A procedure not without risk—not to be undertaken because the doctor is going on vacation.

Jaundice   Accumulation of bile pigments in the blood causing the person to appear yellow. The bile pigment bilirubin forms from the breakdown of red cells and is converted in the liver to a harmless substance excreted through the bile ducts and intestine. In the newborn baby the liver may not be fully functioning, and bilirubin may accumulate causing brain damage. Exchange transfusion is carried out when the blood level of this substance is likely to harm the baby.

Labia   The labia majora and the labia minora are the folds of skin on either side of the entrance of the vagina. They vary considerably in size in different people.

Labor   As it says, hard work! The process of expelling the baby from the uterus by contractions of the thick, strong uterine muscle.

Lactation   The period during which the breasts are producing milk.

Ligaments   Bands of firm fibrous tissue that support organs and hold together bones and joints. They become relaxed during pregnancy to enable the pelvis to be more expansile during labor. Other ligaments may relax, too, causing backache. Physiotherapy assists the return of ligaments and muscles to normal after birth.

Liquor   Amniotic fluid.

Lochia   The discharge that occurs for several weeks after the birth of a baby, at first bloodstained, later yellowish, not usually offensive.

Lubricants   Jellylike medicaments used for vaginal and rectal examination by doctor or nurse to ensure that the gloved finger causes no discomfort from friction in entering the passages. Similar water-soluble lubricants are very useful during sexual intercourse, enabling better timing and synchronizing of sexual climax.

Meconium   The black or greenish-black substance passed from the baby's bowel during the first few days after birth. It contains bile pigments and waste tissue and chemical substances and secretions.

Midstream specimen   Collection of a specimen of urine while it is being passed, to detect infection of the urinary tract. The most reliable way of collecting a specimen for bacteriological examination is to wash the external genitalia, discard the first stream of urine, then collect some into a sterile container while the urine is still flowing.

Midwife   A nurse with special training in the management of labor and care of mother and child during the prenatal period and postnatal period. Most midwives in Australia are trained nurses who have taken additional midwifery training; in some countries a nurse may just train in midwifery.

Molding   Shaping of the baby's head as it passes through the pelvis and rotates to make the passage easier. Because of the number of bones in the skull and their soft state, this can occur gradually without harming the baby.

Mucus   There are many mucous-secreting glands through the body that produce clear, slippery, gelatinous-type material to lubricate body surfaces. Most lining tissues (as in bowel, nose, and throat, bronchial tubes, and cervix and vagina) have glands that secrete mucus.

Neonatal   Newborn, statistically the first twenty-eight days of life.

Nipple   Teat, part of the breast taken into the baby's mouth with the areola during suckling. An artificial teat through which an infant sucks milk from a nursing bottle.

Obstetrician   A physician who treats the mother and baby during pregnancy and labor. The qualifications of the obstetrician are the same as those of the gynecologist.

Occipital bone   The bone making up the base of the skull.

Orgasm   Sexual climax.

Ovulation   Production of a mature ovum with its discharge into the abdominal cavity from the ovary; an operation delicately controlled by nature that can now be controlled artificially.

Oxytocin   The natural hormone stored in the posterior part of the pituitary gland causing contraction of the uterine muscle in labor and of the myoepithelial cells surrounding milk-secreting glands and causing the let-down of milk. Also secreted in sexual intercourse.

Pelvis The strong bony framework made of two hipbones and the sacrum (lower part of spine). The baby has to pass through the central cavity during labor.

Perineum The external area that includes the anus and vulva.

Pethidine A pain-relieving drug often given by injection during the first stage of labor.

Pituitary An endocrine gland about the size of a large pea situated at the base of the brain and involved in the control of all other endocrine glands. It was know as "the conductor of the endocrine orchestra" until it was discovered that the hypothalamus contained releasing factors.

Placenta Afterbirth, organ that conveys nutrition to the developing child and removes waste to the mother's bloodstream.

Placenta previa The situation that occurs when the placenta wholly or partially lies across the cervix. Caesarean section is necessary to deliver the baby safely, and bleeding during pregnancy may be the first indication that this is the problem.

Postmature When a pregnancy has exceeded the expected duration by two weeks it is regarded as prolonged and the baby as postmature.

PPH Postpartum hemorrhage, bleeding occurring after the delivery of the baby. This can be severe but is easily controlled in a hospital; it is the main risk the mother faces if she has a baby at home.

PR Examination by the rectum. A gloved finger is inserted into the rectum to feel the extent to which the cervix has opened.

Progesterone Female sex hormone mainly produced in the ovary, in the second half of the menstrual cycle, and in the placenta.

Pudendal block Local anesthetic given by injection through the vaginal wall or perineum to remove sensation in the perineum. A very safe procedure.

Puerperium The period of recovery following the birth of the baby.

Quickening The sensation of feeling the first movements of the developing child.

Rectum The lower part of the bowel.

Scrotum The external sac that contains the testis.

Semen The fluid containing sperm and secretions from other glands of the male reproductive system that is ejaculated at orgasm.

Smear test   Papanicolaou smear, cyto test, the examination of cells of the cervix mainly for detection of cancer. Formerly this was considered necessary only for middle-aged women; but with the increase in cancer of the cervix, it is now considered desirable in all women over twenty-five, particularly those who have had intercourse in their early teens.

Sphincter   Circular muscle that surrounds the entrance or exit to some parts of the body; e.g., anal sphincter.

Stillbirth   Baby born dead, i.e., without breathing.

Term   Due date.

Thrombosis   Occurrence of blood clot in veins, more likely to occur in pregnancy or after delivery, particularly in women with varicose veins. It can have serious complications and support hose must be worn for a prolonged period, preferably years, after such a thrombosis has occurred.

Thrush   A common infection of the vagina and cervix during pregnancy caused by Monilia *(Candida albicans)* and often transmitted to the baby. It is not serious, but is very irritating. Effective treatment is available.

Toxemia   A condition that can occur in pregnancy when there is a rise in blood pressure, protein in the urine, and swelling. It can endanger the life of mother and baby if not recognized early and treated. Adequate prenatal supervision makes this possible.

Trilene   An inhalation anesthetic used for delivery, though not used much now due to side effects.

Umbilicus   Navel, belly button, the site of attachment of the umbilical vessels that convey blood from the placenta, carrying food and oxygen to the baby in the uterus. These vessels are clamped at birth and drop off after about five days. The beauty of the resultant navel has nothing to do with the ability of the doctor, and some navels are more prominent than others.

Ureter   Tube conveying urine from kidney to bladder.

Urethra   Tube conveying urine from bladder out of the body.

Vacuum extraction   A method of exerting traction on the baby's head to assist in delivery, as an alternative to forceps, by creating a vacuum with suction.

Vagina Entrance to female genitalia internally.

Vas deferens The tube through which the sperm pass in the male from testis to seminal vesicles where they are stored. This tube is cut in the operation of vasectomy.

Vulva External entrance to the vagina.

Bibliography

Attempting to draw up a bibliography, I soon realized that it was an impossible task to list the mass of references to individual articles that fill my study to overflowing. I also saw no reason to recommend that any of my readers should have to wade through all I had to read under the label of sexual freedom. I found that some of the most valuable books such as the World Health Organization Public Health Papers contained articles by the world authorities, and that these gave a list of references, many of which I had used and therefore do not need to list separately.

After I had completed my book and was adding the final touches, an excellent book for teachers becoming involved in family life education came into my hands. *Human Sexual Expression*, by Benjamin Kogan. I found it embarrassing but gratifying to see that most of my references, and in fact many of the quotes I had selected for inclusion in my book, had been used in this book; maybe there has been some similar thinking by two people who care about the welfare of children, though I naturally do not agree with all the observations and my female sex has probably made me more emotional and less neutral. Another book I read at the same time was *The Female Woman*, by Arianna Stassinopoulos, and I hope that all women interested in raising the status of women will read this book.

It is also not possible to list the journals that constantly proceed through this house. Here, the *Medical Journal of Australia*, the *British*

Medical Journal, the *Lancet* make their regular appearance on subscription; medical libraries provide the British and American pediatric and obstetric journals; the valuable journals that produce abstracts, such as *Modern Medicine,* the *Psychiatric Spectator, Pediatric Currents,* Maternity Center Association *Briefs,* present impartial reports at very frequent intervals. So it is very unlikely that I have missed any scientific discoveries of importance.

One of the most valuable magazines I have received constantly during the past twenty years has been the *Child Family Digest* (USA) that became *Child and Family,* established by Charlotte Aiken and her husband as a memorial to the son they lost in the war.

AINSWORTH, MARY D., "The Effects of Maternal Deprivation: A review of findings and controversy in the context of research strategy," in *Reassessment of the Effects of Deprivation of Maternal Care.* Public Health Papers, No. 14, World Health Organization, Geneva, 1962.

BARCLAY, WILLIAM, *Ethics in a Permissive Society.* Fontana, London, 1971.

BAUMGARTNER, LEONA, "Women in Industry—Their Children," in Medical Women's International Association, 12th International Congress (Melbourne).

BEAUVOIR, SIMONE DE, *The Second Sex* (translated H. M. Parshley). Rev. ed. Cape, London, 1968.

BERNE, ERIC, *Games People Play.* Grove, New York, 1964.

BILLER, HENRY B., and MEREDITH, DENNIS, *Father Power.* David McKay, New York, 1975.

BOWLBY, JOHN, *Attachment.* Basic Books, New York, 1977.

———, *Maternal Care and Mental Health.* Monograph Series, No. 2, World Health Organization, Geneva, 1951.

BRANT, HERBERT, and BRANT, MARGARET, *A Dictionary of Pregnancy, Childbirth and Contraception.* Nelson, London, 1971.

BRONFENBRENNER, URIE, "The Origins of Alienation," *in Scientific American,* August 1974.

CLINEBELL, HOWARD J., and CLINEBELL, CHARLOTTE H., *The Intimate Marriage.* Harper & Row, New York, 1970.

CONWAY, R., *The Great Australian Stupor: An interpretation of the Australian way of life.* Sun Books, Melbourne, 1971.

DAVIS, MAXINE, *Sexual Responsibility in Marriage.* Fontana, London, 1967.

DUVALL, EVELYN MILLIS, *Why Wait Till Marriage.* Hale, New York, 1965.

ERIKSON, ERIK, *Childhood and Society*. Norton, New York, 1964.

FISHER, SEYMOUR, *Understanding the Female Orgasm*. Basic Books, New York, 1973.

FRIEDAN, BETTY, *The Feminine Mystique*. 2nd ed. Norton, New York, 1974.

FROMM, ERICH, *The Art of Loving*. Harper & Row, New York, 1974.

GERSH, MARVIN J., *How to Raise Children at Home in Your Spare Time*. Stein & Day, New York, 1973.

GESELL, ARNOLD, and ILG, FRANCES L., *Infant and Child in the Culture of Today*. Harper & Bros., New York, 1943.

GLASSER, WILLIAM, *Reality Therapy*. Harper & Row, New York, 1965.

GOLDSTEIN, JOSEPH, FREUD, ANNA, and SOLNIT, ALBERT, *Beyond the Best Interests of the Child*. Free Press, New York, 1973.

GOULD, JONATHAN, ed., *The Prevention of Damaging Stress in Children*. Churchill, London, 1968.

GREER, GERMAINE, *The Female Eunuch*. McGraw-Hill, New York, 1971.

HAMILTON, W. J., and MOSSMAN, H. W., *Human Embryology*. 4th ed. Williams & Wilkins, Baltimore, 1972.

HARLOW, ROBERT G., and PRUGH, DANE G., " 'Masked Deprivation' in Infants and Young Children," in *Reassessment of the Effects of Deprivation of Maternal Care*. Public Health Papers, No. 14, World Health Organization. Geneva, 1962.

HEMMING, JAMES, *Individual Morality*. Nelson, London, 1969.

HILLIARD, MARION, *A Woman Doctor Looks at Love and Life*. Macmillan, London, 1958.

HOLBROOK, DAVID, *Sex and Dehumanization*. Pitman, London, 1972.

HUXLEY, JULIAN, ed., *The Humanist Frame* (essays). Allen & Unwin, London, 1961.

ILLINGWORTH, RONALD, and ILLINGWORTH, CYNTHIA, *Babies and Young Children*. 5th rev. ed. Churchill, London, 1972.

INTERNATIONAL PAEDIATRIC ASSOCIATION, *Proceedings of the International Congress of Paediatrics*, 1971.

ISBISTER, CLAIR, *Preparing for Motherhood*. Angus & Robertson, Sydney, 1963.

_____, *Mommy, I Feel Sick*. Hawthorn, New York, 1978.

_____, *Birth, Infancy and Childhood*. 2nd ed. Farleigh Press, Sydney, 1971.

_____, "The Family Past, Present and Future." *Medical Journal of Australia*, 14 April 1973, pp. 762–4.

_____, "Family Liberation." *Medical Journal of Australia*, 4 January 1975, pp. 5–9.

———, "The Adopted Child and His Parents." *Medical Journal of Australia*, 9 June 1973, pp. 1158–61.

———, "Mother on the Watch," in *Health Begins at Home*. 25th Anniversary World Health Organization Assembly, Geneva, 1973.

JAMES, MURIEL, and JONGEWARD, DOROTHY, *Born to Win*. Addison-Wesley, Reading, Mass., 1971.

KINSEY, ALFRED C., et al., *Sexual Behaviour in the Human Male*. Saunders, Philadelphia, 1948.

———, *Sexual Behaviour in the Human Female*. Saunders, Philadelphia, 1953.

KOGAN, B. A., *Human Sexual Expression*. Harcourt Brace Jovanovich, New York, 1973.

KORNITZER, M., *Adoption and Family Life*. Putnam, London, 1968.

KRUPINSKI, JERZY, and STOLLER, ALAN, eds., *The Family in Australia*. Pergamon Press, Rushcutters Bay, 1974.

LA LECHE LEAGUE INTERNATIONAL, *The Womanly Art of Breastfeeding*. La Leche League International, Franklin Park, Ill., 1963.

LAYCOCK, S. R., *Family Living and Sex Education*. Baxter, Toronto, 1967.

LEBOVICI, S., "A Child Psychiatrist on Children in Day Care Centres," in *Care of Children in Day Centres*. Public Health Papers, No. 24, World Health Organization, Geneva, 1964.

LEWIS, C. S., *The Four Loves*. Harcourt Brace Jovanovich, New York, 1971.

MacKEITH, RONALD, and WOOD, CHRISTOPHER, *Infant Feeding and Feeding Difficulties*. 4th ed. Churchill, London, 1971.

MAKARENKO, A. S., *Collective Family*. Peter Smith, Gloucester, Mass., 1964.

MASTERS, W. H., and JOHNSON, V. E., *Human Sexual Inadequacy*. Little, Brown, Boston, 1970.

MAY, ROLLO, *Love and Will*. Norton, New York, 1969.

MEAD, MARGARET, "A Cultural Anthropological Approach to Maternal Deprivation", in *Deprivation of Maternal Care*. Public Health Papers, No. 14, World Health Organization, Geneva, 1962.

MEDICAL WOMEN'S INTERNATIONAL ASSOCIATION, 12th International Congress (Melbourne), *The Health of Women in Industry: Scientific Papers*, 1970.

MIDDLEMORE, MERELL P. *The Nursing Couple*. Cassell, London, 1945.

MILLETT, KATE, *Sexual Politics*. Doubleday, New York, 1970.

MOTULSKY, A. G., and LENZ, W., eds., *Birth Defects*. Summary of 4th International Conference on Birth Defects (Vienna, 1973). Excerpta Medica, Amsterdam, 1974.

NATIONAL CHILDREN'S BUREAU, LONDON, *Born Illegitimate: Social and educational implications.* National Foundation for Educational Research in England and Wales, Slough, 1971.

NEWTON, NILES, *Maternal Emotions.* Psychosomatic Medicine Monographs, Harper & Bros., New York, 1955.

NEWTON, NILES, and MEAD, MARGARET, "Cultural Patterning of Perinatal Behavior," in S.A. Richardson and A.F. Guttmacher, eds., *Childbearing—Its Social and Psychological Aspects.* Williams & Wilkins, Baltimore, 1967.

PACKARD, VANCE, *The Sexual Wilderness.* McKay, New York, 1968.

PARKER, GILLIAN, "Family Patterns of Stress and Distress," in Jonathan Gould, ed., *The Prevention of Damaging Stress in Children.* Churchill, London, 1968.

PHILLIPS, VIRGINIA, *Successful Breast Feeding.* Down Under Publishing, Artarmon, 1974.

POLLAK, M., *Today's Three Year Olds in London.* Heinemann, London, 1972.

POPENOE, PAUL, "What is ahead of Us?" *Family Life*, vol. 33, no. 4, American Institute of Family Relations, Los Angeles, 1973.

READ, GRANTLEY DICK, *Childbirth without Fear: The Principles and Practice of Natural Childbirth.* 2nd ed. Heinemann, London, 1952.

RIBBLE, MARGARET A., *The Rights of Infants.* Columbia University Press, New York, 1953.

ROYAL COLLEGE OF OBSTETRICIANS AND GYNAECOLOGISTS, *Unplanned Pregnancy.* Report of the Working Party. London, 1972.

STASSINOPOULOS, ARIANNA, *The Female Woman.* Dell, New York, 1975.

STOLLER, ALAN, ed., *The Family Today.* Published for Victorian Family Council. Cheshire, Melbourne, 1962.

STORR, ANTHONY, *The Integrity of the Personality.* Atheneum, New York, 1961.

SUTTIE, IAN, *The Origins of Love and Hate.* Penguin, Harmondsworth, 1963.

TAVISTOCK INSTITUTE OF HUMAN RELATIONS, *Determinants of Infant Behaviour.* Proceedings of Tavistock study groups on mother-infant interaction, 1959–65, ed. B. M. Foss. 4 vols, Methuen, London, 1961–9.

TIERNEY, LEN J., "Multiproblem Families," in J. Krupinski and A. Stoller, eds., *The Family in Australia.* Pergamon Press, Rushcutters Bay, 1974.

TOFFLER, A., *Future Shock*. Random House, New York, 1970.

VELLAY, PIERRE, et al., *Childbirth without Pain* (translated from the French by Denise Lloyd). Dutton, New York, 1959.

WILLIAMS, R. H., *To Live and to Die: When, Why and How*. Springer-Verlag, New York, 1973.

WILSON, DONALD P., "Premarital Experience No Help in Sexual Adjustment After Marriage." *Family Life*, vol. 32, no. 5, American Institute of Family Relations, Los Angeles, 1972.

WINNICOTT, D. W., *The Child, the Family and the Outside World*, Penguin, Harmondsworth, 1970.

UNITED STATES DEPARTMENT OF LABOR, WOMEN'S BUREAU, *Who Are the Working Mothers?* 1972.

Index